CARE TECHNOLOGIES FOR AGEING SOCIETIES

Sustainable Care

Series Editors:
Sue Yeandle, University of Sheffield,
Jon Glasby, University of Birmingham,
Jill Manthorpe, King's College London and
Kate Hamblin, University of Sheffield

This series provides novel contributions to understanding care systems, care work and care relationships. Focusing on the concept of 'sustainable care', it makes an innovative and distinctive contribution to understandings of future care challenges and how care arrangements could be made more sustainable.

Available in the Series

Social Care in the UK's Four Nations
Between Two Paradigms
Edited by **Catherine Needham** and **Patrick Hall**

Forthcoming in the Series

Combining Work and Care
Carer Leave and Related Employment Policies in International Context
Edited by **Janet Fast**, **Kate Hamblin** and **Jason Heyes**

Find out more

policy.bristoluniversitypress.co.uk/sustainable-care

For citizens, practitioners and policy makers who imagine better care futures

Contents

Series editor preface

The *Sustainable Care* book series arises from a large grant programme, Sustainable Care: connecting people and systems, delivered by a multidisciplinary partnership of 35 scholars in eight universities, funded by the UK's Economic and Social Research Council. It provides novel, interdisciplinary and internationally informed contributions based on work by linked research teams studying care systems, care work and care relationships.

Our focus is timely and important. The series is presenting the findings from a distinctive programme of new research on social care. Our main aims for the series are that it will make an innovative and distinctive contribution to understandings of future care challenges and how they could be addressed. The series offers new empirical, conceptual and methodological writing, in scholarly but accessible form, aimed to inform and inspire scholars, policy makers, employers, practitioners and citizens interested in care.

The Sustainable Care programme's book series with Policy Press brings together data, practices, systems, structures, narratives and actions relevant to social care, particularly our ageing populations. While much of our subject matter is distinct and specific to the UK's unique policy, demographic, cultural and socio-economic circumstances, it also has clear global relevance. Similar concerns are salient around the world and especially relevant in other advanced welfare states: population ageing is profoundly changing age structures; developments in technology and in healthcare mean more people who are ill or have long-term conditions need support at home; and 'traditional' gendered sources of daily caring labour are dwindling, as levels of female labour force participation rise and family networks become more dispersed. The COVID-19 pandemic has amplified such challenges.

Subject areas, disciplines and themes

The series critically engages with fierce contemporary debates about care infrastructure; divisions of caring labour and the political economy of care; care ethics, rights, recognition and values; care technologies and human–technology interactions; and care relations in intergenerational, emotional, community and familial context. Within its overarching concept, sustainable care, its subject areas span social and welfare policy and systems; family and social gerontology; ageing and disability studies; employment and workforce organisation; diversity (including gender and ethnicity); social work and human resources; migration and mobility; and technology studies.

We all have the potential to benefit from new multidisciplinary work on care that embraces progress in global scholarship on diversity, culture and the uses of technology, and engages with issues of inequality, political economy and the division of labour. These were the distinctive features of our programme and they are highlighted and developed in this book series. We are grateful to all who have contributed as researchers, programme administrators and research participants, to our funders, our advisory group and to members of the public who have engaged with our studies so far. We hope this series of books reflects the quality of their contributions. We thank each book's editors, authors and our publisher for their commitment to spreading ideas, knowledge and experiences.

Jon Glasby, Kate Hamblin,
Jill Manthorpe and
Sue Yeandle

List of figures, tables and boxes

Figures

Tables

Boxes

Notes on contributors

Arlene Astell is Professor at and Director of the Dementia Ageing Technology Engagement (DATE) lab at KITE, University Health Network, Toronto, Canada and Professor of Neurocognitive Diseases at the University of Reading, UK. She is also Senior Scientist at Samsung AI Center, where she leads the Wellbeing Lab. Arlene has more than 20 years of experience developing and evaluating interventions to support people to age as well as possible, including those living with dementia.

Lindy Clemson is Emeritus Professor at The University of Sydney, Australia. She has developed innovative and accessible programmes, underpinned by enabling strategies, so that as we age, we can lead safe and active lives and stay connected with community. Her work is underpinned by recognition that everyone has a right to access evidence-based interventions that meet their needs and to understand their benefit. Internationally, she is in the top ten most published fall prevention trial researchers, and more recently conducted translational research in reablement programmes for people living with dementia. Her work has influenced policy and practice, with Cochrane Reviews and national practice guidelines.

Janet Fast is Professor in the Department of Human Ecology at the University of Alberta, Canada and Co-director of the Research on Aging, Policies, and Practice research programme.

She holds a PhD in family and consumer economics from Cornell University, NY, USA. Major themes of her research are the economics of ageing and the paid and unpaid care work of family members. She is a member of the leadership team of the AGE-WELL National Centres of Excellence, Canada's ageing and technology network.

Kate Hamblin is Senior Research Fellow at the Centre for International Research on Care, Labour and Equalities, University of Sheffield, UK. She leads the Economic and Social Research Council (ESRC) Centre for Care's Digital Care research theme and is a member of the ESRC and Health Foundation-funded Improving Adult Care Together (IMPACT) Implementation Centre leadership team. She joined the University of Sheffield in 2018 to work on the ESRC-funded Sustainable Care programme. Her research has focused on technology and its role in the care of older people with complex needs as well as issues related to employment, including the balance between unpaid care and paid work; self-employment and ageing; and 'active ageing' employment and pension policies.

Andreas Hoff is Professor of Social Gerontology at Zittau/Görlitz University of Applied Sciences and Director of the research institute 'Gesundheit, Altern, Arbeit, Technik' (GAT; English translation: 'Health, Ageing, Labour, Technology'), Germany. His research over the past 25 years focused on family care/informal care in the context of different European welfare states, more specifically on the use and co-creation of assistive technologies in older people's homes and in home care, the reconciliation of employment and family care, as well as intergenerational relations in family, community and society.

Matthew Lariviere is Lecturer in Social Policy at the School for Policy Studies at the University of Bristol, UK. Matthew is a social anthropologist whose research examines digital public policy and public services, the socio-materiality of digital technology and artificial intelligence (AI) within care arrangements and everyday life, and futurities of care and ageing. Matthew is an elected Fellow of the Royal Anthropological Institute of Great Britain and Ireland and Fellow of the Higher Education Association.

Meryl Lovarini is Honorary Senior Lecturer in Occupational Therapy at The University of Sydney, Australia. Her research interests include technology for ageing in place, preventing falls among older adults living in the community and implementation science. She has received over AUD$1.3 million in research funding and has co-authored over 40 peer-reviewed publications.

Kate O'Loughlin is Associate Professor (Honorary) and a health sociologist in the School of Health Sciences, the University of Sydney, Australia and Investigator at the Centre of Excellence in Population Ageing Research. Kate's research focuses on mature-age workforce participation and ageing-related health and care policies. Her current research is in three key areas: the socio-economic and political context of combining paid work and carer responsibilities; attitudes to ageing and age discrimination; and use of technology for ageing in place. Published books/chapters include *Ageing in Australia: Challenges and Opportunities* (2017; co-editors Colette Browning and Hal Kendig), *Older Adults and Digital Technologies* (2019; with Meryl Lovarini and Lindy Clemson) and *Ageing and Health* (2022; editors Alphia Possamai-Inesedy and Peta Cook). Kate is an associate editor of *International Journal of Care and Caring* and *Frontiers in Public Health* (Aging).

Bill Pottharst is Research Associate focusing on human–technology interaction in the joint research transfer project Saxony5 and Laboratory Manager of the Ambient Assisted Living (AAL) Lab at the research institute 'Gesundheit,

Altern, Arbeit, Technik' (GAT; English translation: 'Health, Ageing, Labour, Technology') at Zittau/Görlitz University of Applied Sciences, Germany. He received his doctorate in 2021 and published the book *Generation, Ungleichheit, Technik – Technikkompetenz im höheren Lebensalter* ('Generation, Inequality, Technology – Technological Competence in Older Age'). His research over the past eight years focused on human–technology interaction, with a specific focus on assistive technologies for older people, in their homes as well as in the workplace, as well as research on the transfer of scientific knowledge into society.

Tomoko Wakui is Research Fellow at the Tokyo Metropolitan Institute of Gerontology, Japan. Her research interests include social policy, gerontology, family studies, caring and geriatric psychiatry.

James Wright is Research Associate at The Alan Turing Institute, the UK's national institute for data science and AI. He received his PhD in anthropology and science and technology studies (STS) from the University of Hong Kong, China in 2018. His research interests include the development and use of robots, AI and other digital technologies for elder care; his current project, PATH-AI, focuses on AI ethics and governance in the UK and Japan. His first book, entitled *Robots Won't Save Japan: An Ethnography of Eldercare Automation*, was published in early 2023 by Cornell University Press.

Acknowledgements

The editors gratefully acknowledge the support of the (UK) Economic and Social Research Council (ESRC) for the Sustainable Care: connecting people and systems programme (grant reference: ES/P009255/1, 2017–21, principal investigator: Sue Yeandle, University of Sheffield) and Sustainable Care Innovation Fellowship: accelerating implementation and uptake of new technologies to support ageing in place (grant reference: ES/S002049/1, 2018–21, principal investigator: Matthew Lariviere).

ONE

Care technologies for ageing societies: setting the scene

Kate Hamblin and Matthew Lariviere

Technology in policy discourses is frequently cited as pivotal for ameliorating the global 'crisis' in care, delivering positive outcomes, and is increasingly part of care provision and arrangements across the world. This Policy Press Short will explore how, in different national contexts, technology is being deployed to contribute to the sustainability of care relationships, arrangements and services, and the achievement of well-being outcomes for older people.

Our contributors examine technology policy, practice and research evidence from five countries across Europe, Oceania, North America and Asia. The countries selected – Australia, Canada, England, Germany and Japan – all face challenges to the sustainability of care provision due to major demographic changes, such as increased longevity and falling fertility, amplifying demand for quality care services. In all the countries included, technology is increasingly being proposed as a potential means to address challenges related to the shortages in long-term care (LTC) provision, both in terms of resources and the care workforce. This book explores how these countries have integrated technology into their care systems and services, and examines evidence related to outcomes for older people, family carers and care provision.

The countries selected for comparison are unified in their experiences of ageing populations and systemic shifts towards more 'marketised' approaches to care provision. However, in relation to care, the selected countries also have different policy legacies and approaches that shape and channel reform in particular directions. In line with Hantrais and Mangen's (1996: 1–2) assertion that 'a study can be said to be cross-national and comparative if one or more units in two or more societies, cultures and countries are compared in respect of the same concepts and concerning the systematic analysis of phenomena, usually with the intention of explaining them and generalising from them', the comparison provided here will extend this framework to explore technology within care provision. This volume focuses on how nations with different policy contexts, but facing similar demographic pressures, may appear to move in parallel directions in their policy and practice regarding technologies in care services and provision. Such an approach does not make any claims about causal mechanisms; instead, we seek to highlight key points of convergence and divergence across the five selected countries and identify areas for cross-national learning. Our aim is, therefore, to examine the role of technology within these varied systems of care provision that all face similar pressures around their sustainability, and in doing so, hope insights will specify potential ways forward for academics, policy makers and other stakeholders in this field.

Cross-national policy and practice comparisons are challenging, particularly due to the way key concepts 'translate' (or not) across different contexts. Sartori (1970) warns against the perils of 'concept stretching', whereby a term is broadened to be applicable to so many contexts, it loses all coherence and contextually situated meaning. As such, conceptualisation should be done with care to combat conceptual vagueness and an inconsistency across contexts (Hopkin, 2002), but also to avoid essentially becoming meaningless in practice. This introductory chapter therefore begins by defining key concepts that are the substantive focus of the volume: care, technology and sustainability. It then describes the selection of the five country cases to follow in Chapters 2–6, before closing with a short overview of each chapter.

Key concepts

Care

Care has been argued to be a challenging concept, with Daly (2021) highlighting that the lack of a single clear definition has resulted in the development of varied terminology, with, for example, 'social care' and 'long-term care' used interchangeably. For Daly, it is apparent that while authors may use the term 'care', they are not always implicitly defining the concept in the same way. For this reason, we outline here our approach that applies across all chapters in this volume, mindful that we need to provide sufficient room to accommodate national specificity while not tipping over into 'concept stretching'.

Our work builds on the diverse approaches to conceptualising care in past social science and social policy research. Daly (2021) observes care was 'discovered' around 30–40 years ago when what had been seen as a mundane and 'natural' phenomenon began to be explored in research examining areas related to the private sphere of the family and women's roles within, and then also the public sphere of policies and provision for those needing support. In her work, Daly delineates four main literatures with differing conceptualisations of care: '1) care as labour and value orientation; 2) care as a component of welfare state policy; 3) care in the context of the organization and effectiveness of service provision; 4) care as embedded in global processes' (p 109).

This volume draws on several of these literatures. Due to its focus on national policies as the unit of analyses, we touch on the 'care as labour' tradition, centred on activities to support another person viewed as 'care' (unpaid, kin-based work) or as (paid) 'care work' (Graham, 1983; Ungerson, 1983; Bond, 1992). Care in this tradition has also been connected to an ethical responsibility to support the well-being of others, via an 'ethics of care', based on the caregiver's empathy (Gilligan, 1982) and on attentiveness, responsibility, competence and responsiveness to the care receiver (Tronto, 1993; Tronto, 2017). More recent scholarship has focused on 'care as a moral experience' that evokes sensibilities of compassion, respect and love, which is relational, reciprocal and facilitated through touch and co-presence (Kleinman, 2012; Kleinman, 2015; Kleinman, 2017). This tradition, therefore, could be argued to have focused attention on the importance of care and care provision, both as a potential site of inequality but also as an essential part of the human experience (Tronto, 1993). The fourth tradition, exploring how care is embedded in global processes, returns to these discussions of inequalities and power by exploring issues related to global care chains and care across borders (Yeates, 2012; Michel and Peng, 2017).

The second and third of the literatures identified by Daly narrow the focus of analysis to national policies (often as part of cross-national comparisons) or specific policy interventions. The second tradition in Daly's work with which this volume aligns most closely focuses on how welfare states and care interact, with the former defining the parameters of what types of activities are worthy of policy action and intervention. Drawing on this literature, in its exploration of care technologies provided by welfare states, this volume characterises care as 'a domain of need and exigency' (Daly, 2021: 111) and 'ground their conceptualization in the practice of care' (p 113). This tradition is closely linked to the third broad group of literatures, which Daly argued focuses on specific interventions and evaluating the degree to which they can be considered to deliver care-related outcomes. We also touch on this tradition in our approach, bringing in research evidence from each country related to the effectiveness or adequacy of national policies related to technologies within and for care.

Daly, reflecting on these traditions, defines care in a way that encompasses care as both policy and practice but also acknowledges its centrality to human relations. We therefore use Daly's definition to ground our comparative analysis in this book, defining care as 'a vital sphere of human engagement and welfare-related activity focused on practices oriented to meeting perceived need' (2021: 113).

Technology

For this volume, we again aim to provide a definition of technology in relation to care that has sufficient specificity to allow for comparison between countries, while at the same time not imposing a particularly Anglo-centric approach to the concept. Broadly, our focus is on technologies – devices, systems and associated services representing the 'application of scientific knowledge for practical purposes' (Stevenson, 2010) – that have been provided either directly or funded through public care services to facilitate the provision of care or 'human engagement and welfare-related activity focused on practices oriented to meeting perceived need' (Daly, 2021: 113). This gives space to the authors of the chapters to discuss the context-specific ways different types of technologies have been brought into policy and practice, and to bring in different, nationally applicable terms used to describe technologies as related to care. For example, there are discussions of 'telecare', 'technology-enabled care' and, more recently, 'care tech' (DHSC, 2021) in England, 'assistive technologies' in Germany and Australia, and 'technologies' more broadly in Canada, all aimed at meeting needs related to care.

In adopting an approach to defining technology that is grounded in policy and practice, we aim to avoid 'technologically deterministic' and reductive discourses, underplaying the constructed and constructive nature of technology (Holloway and Valentine, 2003). Technologies do not emerge organically and are fundamentally political and social (Ihde, 1993; Custer, 1995; Mackenzie and Wajcman, 1999; Ihde and Selinger, 2003); our contributors explore the policy drivers behind particular approaches to the use of technologies in care provision and practice.

Sustainability

The United Nation's Sustainable Development Goals are often used to underpin discussions and definitions of sustainability. The Sustainable Development Goals aim to create a balance between economic, social and environmental sustainability, with consideration of the long term and implications for future generations. However, the focus of much policy discourse globally has been on the economic sustainability of LTC arrangements, particularly in a context of population ageing, and in turn the use of technology in care systems has been presented as a means to save costs. Population ageing, while in part the result of advances in health and welfare programmes that have increased longevity, can create additional pressure on care arrangements and provision. Globally, in 2020, there were 727 million people aged 65 years or over and this number is projected to more than double, reaching over 1.5 billion by 2050. In 2020, the share of the population aged 65 or over was 9.3 per cent; by 2050, it is projected to be 16.0 per cent (UNDESA, 2020).

However, we highlight that sustainability can be defined more broadly than in purely economic terms, applying the idea of a 'triple bottom-line' to social care in order to 'seek to have a system that is not only financially sustainable, but also minimises adverse impacts on society and on the natural environment, which could jeopardise the ability of future generations to meet their health and social care needs' (Naylor and Appleby, 2012: 2). Social sustainability has been linked to the concept of well-being in discussions of care, insofar as it has been argued 'sustainable care … requires the wellbeing of the different actors in care arrangements' (Keating et al, 2021: 2). Care arrangements that unduly burden or damage the well-being of those either receiving or providing care in a paid or unpaid capacity can therefore be argued to be unsustainable. Well-being in turn has been conceptualised as a multifaceted concept, with three dimensions: the material (what a person has), the relational (their relationships with others) and the subjective (how they feel) (McGregor, 2018). The question is therefore whether technologies in care provision and arrangements can protect or enhance well-being of the various actors and, in so doing, contribute to sustainable care. In addition, the application of technologies to care also raises issues of ecological sustainability in terms of the environmental impact of their production and disposal.

Countries for comparison

Part of the rationale for selecting the countries of Australia, Canada, Germany, England and Japan is grounded in the care regime literature (Bettio and Plantenga, 2004) but also to demographic developments in these nations, in line with Sartori's argument: '[t]he comparisons in which we sensibly and actually engage are thus those between entities whose attributes are in part shared (similar) and in part non-shared (and thus, we say, incomparable)' (1994: 17). In terms of the similarities between these nations, countries in Europe, Asia, North America and Oceania are all undergoing demographic ageing. Europe is currently the most aged continent, with one fifth of its population (20.8 per cent) aged over 65 in 2021 (Eurostat, 2021). In England, 18.4 per cent of the population were over 65 in 2021 (ONS, 2022). East and South East Asia is the most rapidly ageing area, with the population aged 65 years or over almost doubling from 6 per cent in 1990 to 11 per cent in 2019 (UNDESA, 2019). In Japan, 28.7 per cent of the population were 65 or older and the country was also home to a record 80,000 centenarians in 2020 (European Parliament, 2020). Similarly, Australia is also undergoing population ageing, with 16 per cent of the population aged 65 or older in 2020 (4.2 million; AIHW, 2021). In Canada, 18.5 per cent of the population in 2021 was aged 65 and older (Statistics Canada, 2022).

There is also an argument that in response to the challenges related to population ageing, these countries are converging on similar policy solutions, despite very different policy histories. Peng and Yeandle (2017) argue cross-national policy learning has led to the adoption of long-term care insurance (LTCI) policies in some East Asian nations, based on the German LTCI policy, which provides cash allowances or care services. There has also been an increase in the marketisation of social care across Europe and East Asia, 'as many governments attempt to privatize systems that were hitherto publicly funded or to further reinforce the private market role in the provision of care' (Peng and Yeandle, 2017: 3). England provides personal budgets to allow the purchase of care on the private market (subject to means- and needs-test assessments), and Australia moved to a similar system to provide 'home care packages' in 2013. In Japan, the quasi-market system is strictly regulated by the government and care is delivered through both public and private sectors (Peng and Yeandle, 2017). In many Canadian provinces, people may opt for 'self-managed care' where they receive a monthly allowance to use towards the costs of their care (Spalding et al, 2006).

While these selected countries are facing similar challenges to the sustainability of their welfare systems and appear to be shifting to a marketised model of care provision, there remain important differences in their policy approaches, reflecting the importance of policy, historical and institutional contexts (Peng and Yeandle, 2017: 1–2). These differing policy approaches are underscored by the care regime literature. This literature highlighted that research developing welfare typologies of national social policies focused on the labour market and the ability of individuals to withdraw from it (Esping-Andersen, 1990), and in so doing eliding the issue of unpaid work within the private sphere of the home.[1] As such, 'decommodified' women were often engaged in unpaid care work (Pfau-Effinger, 2005a, b); the care regime literature, therefore, examines the extent to which welfare provision offers opportunity for 'defamilialisation', or 'the degree to which individual adults can uphold a socially acceptable standard of living, independently of family relationships, either through paid work or through the social security system' (Lister, 1994: 37). Bettio and Plantenga (2004) proposed that the level of care or degree of defamilialisation provided by the state varies according to cultural and political legacies, with care organised to reflect cultural attitudes about the family. In some nations, care is considered a private matter for the family and, therefore, policy treats it as such. In other countries, however, care is provided by the state or market to allow both sexes to engage in paid employment. The care regime literature emphasises that the varying role states play in providing care has implications either for the family or the market as the provider of care.

The care regime literature has produced several examples of typologies that classify nations according to the provision of care for either children or dependent adults (or both), though there is no universally accepted typology (Peng and Yeandle, 2017). Studies have also highlighted the importance of disentangling policies for childcare from care for adults when classifying nations into care regimes (Bettio and Plantenga, 2004). Typically, these models classified England (as part of the United Kingdom) as part of a liberal, male breadwinner regime where the state provided care, services and allowances for children while for older adults, the family has the primary responsibility for care (Bettio and

Plantenga, 2004). Similarly, in Germany, the family has had the responsibility for the provision of care, following the principle of 'subsidiarity', whereby the state provision was minimal so as not to 'crowd out' the family (Tester, 1994). More recent analyses that have focused on European countries have observed convergence towards the trend discussed above towards marketisation or the increased use of private care services, with a particular focus on supporting, without replacing, family care and a shift to 'care in the community' and away from residential or institutional care for older people (Bettio and Verashcaghina, 2009).

Looking outside of Europe, both welfare and care regime literatures have often placed Australia and Canada alongside the UK/England as part of a 'liberal' regime, with the state's role largely limited to providing targeted assistance to those who are least well-off. However, it is argued they have quite distinct histories of care provision that set them apart from England (Brennan et al, 2012). Australia has a strong tradition of delivering care through publicly subsidised non-profit organisations whereas in England, local authorities provided much of the care for older people until the 1990s, where there was a shift to the marketisation or 'contracting out' to other providers (private and not-for-profit). In Canada, LTC is assigned to provinces and territories as part of the federal system of government but there are core services as they are supplied in all jurisdictions, including LTC institutions, palliative care, respite care, rehabilitation services such as physiotherapy and occupational therapy, domestic help and personal care services. Whereas England, which also relies on means testing, is characterised as having a strict system with 'safety net' provision, Canada is classed alongside nations where 'the majority of means tests are not very restrictive, meaning that the public cost share does not vary much between people with high and low income or assets' (Muir, 2017: 27). However, 75 per cent of all care is provided by informal (largely family) carers in Canada (Stall, 2019).

The inclusion of an East Asian nation in this book also enhances our cross-national comparison. Japan exhibits a strong reliance on families to provide care but has also seen a more active involvement of the state in the provision of care (supplemented by the market and community) than other East Asian nations, where the state's role is more limited and thus there is greater reliance on the market and community (Chan et al, 2011). Though care for older adults was seen historically as family responsibility, Japan has introduced a public social care system. The rapid ageing of the population and the rising cost of hospital care following the introduction of free medical care for older people in 1973 prompted the government to introduce the 'Gold Plan' public social care system for older people in 1989, including a means-tested supplementary public service delivered by local governments to provide community-based care for older adults. As family formations continued to change in the 1990s with rising numbers of women in employment and therefore unable to provide care for parents and parents-in-law, Japan introduced a similar scheme to Germany's LTCI that provides universal care to those over the age of 65 and aged 40–64 with age-related disabilities. The scheme, funded by a compulsory social insurance system for all citizens over the age of 40, differs from Germany's in that it is needs-tested rather than means-tested, but has been described as a 'quasi-market model' (Peng and Yeandle, 2017).

Structure of this volume

This volume opens with the chapter on technology and care provision in England. James Wright and co-editor Kate Hamblin begin by briefly setting out the context of the English 'adult social care' system, including the situation regarding funding and policy, key statistics, and the hopes invested by the government and local authorities in the use of technology to cut costs while improving the quality of life of older people. The analysis of the use of technology in social care is divided into three sections: 1. digital technologies intended to facilitate the delivery of care, including telecare, telemedicine, apps and robotics; 2. technological infrastructure, including the 'digital switchover', broadband and 4G/5G telecommunication networks; and 3. data and information, including the emergent use of digital care management systems, algorithms and artificial intelligence. In each case, key related policies and funding schemes are described and the introduction and state of actual use of different technologies assessed. The chapter concludes by setting out the key policy challenges facing the testing and implementation of technology in England's care sector.

Meryl Lovarini, Kate O'Loughlin and Lindy Clemson then explore the use of technologies in care provision in Australia. This chapter provides an overview of Australia's policy framework related to care for older people and 'ageing in place', outlines the role of technologies in supporting older people to remain in community settings, and reports on research studies identifying issues related to knowledge and use of technology. The authors make recommendations for advancing research along with strategies for care professionals to support older adults' use of assistive/digital technologies.

In the chapter focused on Germany, Andreas Hoff and Bill Pottharst explore the aspirations of governments that technologies – specifically assistive technologies – will meet some of the challenges related to the ageing population. This chapter first outlines the structure of social care provision in Germany, including some key statistics. The central section critically reviews principles, policy and practice of technology use in social care provision, concluding with a brief summary of relevant research evidence and some recommendations related to greater involvement of older people and their carers in the development of technologies for use in care arrangements and systems.

Arlene Astell and Janet Fast examine policy and practice in Canada, where the lack of a legislated mandate for care provision and federated government structure (a central federal government and 13 semi-autonomous provincial/territorial governments) results in overlapping jurisdiction over, and substantial variability in, care services to the extent that it could be argued this nation lacks a social care 'system'. The authors describe the nature of social care in Canada; what is delivered (and not delivered), by whom and how, in the context of overlapping jurisdictions; and the role of technology in this complex setting.

In the chapter focused on Japan, Tomoko Wakui highlights the country's rapid population ageing and associated challenges, including the struggle to maintain people's quality of life while sustaining the social care system to support older adults, as well as those with care needs. The declining birth rate has led to smaller household structures, and the financial burden of maintaining the public LTC and medical insurance programmes on society has increased gradually. It is in this context that Japan is introducing technologies into care settings, with the hope of securing the sustainability of LTC arrangements.

Our volume then concludes with a chapter that explores the areas of divergence and convergence in policy, practice and evidence from the five nations. Drawing on the insights from these countries, we close with recommendations related to the use of technology in care provision and arrangements for policy makers, practitioners and researchers from academia and industry.

Note

1 However, it is important to highlight that the 'use of regime typologies involves generalisation from actual policies and real-life arrangements, which can result in glossing over internal differences within actual national policy regimes … a finer grained analysis … brings out important intra- as well as inter-regime differences' (Mahon et al, 2012: 421).

References

Australian Institute of Health and Welfare [AIHW]. (2021) 'Older Australia at a glance'. Web report. Available at: https://www.aihw.gov.au/reports/older-people/older-australia-at-a-glance/contents/summary [accessed 01.08.22].

Bettio, F. and Plantenga, J. (2004) 'Comparing care regimes in Europe', *Feminist Economics*, 10(1): 85–113.

Bettio, S. and Verashchagina, A. (2009) 'Fiscal system and female employment in Europe'. European Commission. Directorate General for Employment, Social Affairs and Equal Opportunities, EU: Luxembourg.

Bond, J. (1992) 'The politics of caregiving: the professionalisation of informal care', *Ageing and Society*, 12(1): 5–21.

Brennan, D., Cass, B., Himmelweit, S. and Szebehely, M. (2012) 'The marketisation of care: rationales and consequences in Nordic and liberal care regimes', *Journal of European Social Policy*, 22(4): 377–391.

Chan, R.K.H., Soma, N. and Yamashita, J. (2011) 'Care regimes and responses: East Asian experiences compared', *Journal of Comparative Social Welfare*, 27(2): 175–186.

Custer, R.L. (1995) 'Examining the dimensions of technology', *International Journal of Technology and Design Education*, 5(3): 219–244.

Daly, M. (2021) 'The concept of care: insights, challenges and research avenues in COVID-19 times', *Journal of European Social Policy*, 31(1): 108–118.

Department of Health and Social Care [DHSC]. (2021) 'People at the heart of care: adult social care reform'. London: DHSC.

Esping-Andersen, G. (1990) *The Three Worlds of Welfare Capitalism*, Princeton, New Jersey: Princeton University Press.

European Parliament. (2020) 'Japan's ageing society'. Briefing: continental democracies. Available at: https://www.europarl.europa.eu/RegData/etudes/BRIE/2020/659419/EPRS_BRI(2020)659419_EN.pdf [accessed 18.07.22].

Eurostat. (2021) 'Population structure and ageing'. Available at: https://ec.europa.eu/eurostat/statistics-explained/index.php?title=Population_structure_and_ageing [accessed 18.01.23].

Gilligan, C. (1982) *In A Different Voice: Psychological Theory and Women's Development*, Cambridge, Mass.: Harvard University Press.

Graham, H. (1983) 'Caring: a labour of love', in Finch, J. and Groves, D. (Eds) *A Labour of Love: Women, Work and Caring*, London: Routledge, pp 13–30.

Hantrais, L. and Mangen, S.P. (Eds). (1996) *Cross National Research Methods*, London: Pinter.

Holloway, S.L. and Valentine, G. (2003) *Cyberkids: Children in the Information Age*, London: Routledge.

Hopkin, J. (2002) 'Comparative methods', in Marsh, D. and Stoker, G. (Eds) *Theory and Methods in Political Science* (2nd edition), Basingstoke: Palgrave Macmillan.

Ihde, D. (1993) *Philosophy of Technology*. New York: Paragon House.

Ihde, D. and Selinger E. (2003) *Chasing Technoscience: Matrix of Materiality*. Bloomington, Indiana: Indiana University Press.

Keating, N., McGregor, J.A. and Yeandle, S. (2021) 'Sustainable care: theorising the wellbeing of caregivers to older persons', *International Journal of Care and Caring*, 5(4): 611–630.

Kleinman, A. (2012) 'Caregiving as moral experience', *The Lancet*, 380(9853): 1550–1551.

Kleinman, A. (2015) 'Care: in search of a health agenda', *The Lancet*, 386(9990): 240–241.

Kleinman, A. (2017) 'Presence', *The Lancet*, 389(10088): 2466–2467.

Lister, R. (1994) '"She has other duties": women, citizenship and social security', in Baldwin, S. and Falkingham, J. (Eds) *Social Security and Social Change: New Challenges*, Hemel Hempstead: Harvester Wheatsheaf, pp 31–44.

MacKenzie, D. and Wajcman, J. (Eds). (1999) *The Social Shaping of Technology* (2nd edition), Buckingham: Open University Press.

Mahon, R., Anttonen, A., Bergqvist, C., Brennan, D. and Hobson, B. (2012) 'Convergent care regimes? Childcare arrangements in Australia, Canada, Finland and Sweden', *Journal of European Social Policy*, 22(4): 419–431.

McGregor, J.A. (2018) 'Reconciling universal frameworks and local realities in understanding and measuring wellbeing', in Bache, I. and Scott, K. (Eds) *The Politics of Wellbeing*, Basingstoke: Palgrave Macmillan.

Michel, S. and Peng, I. (2017) *Gender, Migration and the Work of Care*. Cham, Switzerland: Palgrave Macmillan.

Muir, T. (2017) 'Measuring social protection for long-term care', *OECD Health Working Papers*, Paris: OECD Publishing.

Naylor, C. and Appleby, J. (2012) *Sustainable Health and Social Care: Connecting Environmental and Financial Performance*, London: The King's Fund.

Office of National Statistics [ONS]. (2022) 'Population and household estimates, England and Wales: Census 2021'. Available at: https://www.ons.gov.uk/peoplepopulationandcommunity/populationandmigration/populationestimates/bulletins/populationandhouseholdestimatesenglandandwales/census2021 [accessed 20.11.22].

Peng, I. and Yeandle, S.M. (2017) *Eldercare Policies in East Asia and Europe: Mapping Policy Changes and Variations and their Implications*, New York: UN Women Discussion Paper Series, United Nations Entity for Gender Equality and the Empowerment of Women (UN Women).

Pfau-Effinger, B. (2005a) 'Culture and welfare state policies: reflections on a complex interrelation', *Journal of Social Policy*, 34(1): 3–20.

Pfau-Effinger, B. (2005b) 'Welfare state policies and the development of care arrangements', *European Societies*, 7(2): 321–347.

Sartori, G. (1970) 'Concept misformation in comparative politics', *American Political Science Review*, 64: 1033–1053.

Sartori, G. (1994) 'Compare why and how: comparing, miscomparing and the comparative method' in Dogan, M. and Kazancigil, A. (Eds) *Comparing Nations: Concepts, Strategies, Substance*, London: Basil Blackwell, pp 14–34.

Spalding, K., Watkins, J.R. and Williams, A.P. (2006) *Self-Managed Care Programs in Canada: A Report to Health Canada*, Ottawa: Health Canada.

Stall, N. (2019) 'We should care more about caregivers', *Canadian Medical Association Journal*, 191(9): E245–E246.

Statistics Canada. (2022) 'Older adults and population aging statistics'. Available at: https://www.statcan.gc.ca/en/subjects-start/older_adults_and_population_aging [accessed 28.06.22].

Stevenson, A. (Ed). (2010) *Oxford Dictionary of English* (3rd edition), Oxford: Oxford University Press.

Tester, S. (1994) 'Implications of subsidiarity for the care of older people in Germany', *Social Policy and Administration*, 28(3): 251–262.

Tronto, J.C. (1993) 'Beyond gender difference to a theory of care: feminist and interdisciplinary perspectives', in Larrabee, M.J. (Ed) *An Ethics of Care: Feminist and Interdisciplinary Perspectives*, London: Routledge, pp 240–257.

Tronto, J.C. (2017) 'There is an alternative: homines curans and the limits of neoliberalism', *International Journal of Care and Caring*, 1(1): 27–43.

Ungerson, C. (1983) 'Why do women care?', in Finch J. and Groves, D. (Eds) *A Labour of Love: Women, Work and Caring*, London: Routledge.

United Nations Department of Economic and Social Affairs [UNDESA]. (2019) 'World population ageing 2019 highlights', Available at: https://www.un.org/en/development/desa/population/publications/pdf/ageing/WorldPopulationAgeing2019-Highlights.pdf [accessed 29.11.22].

United Nations Department of Economic and Social Affairs. (2020) 'World population ageing 2020 highlights'. Available at: https://www.un.org/development/desa/pd/sites/www.un.org.development.desa.pd/files/undesa_pd-2020_world_population_ageing_highlights.pdf [accessed 28.06.22].

Yeates, N. (2012) 'Global care chains: a state-of-the-art review and future directions in care transnationalization research', *Global Networks*, 12(2): 135–154.

TWO

Technology and adult social care in England

James Wright and Kate Hamblin

Social care: policy, debates and evidence in England

The structure of social care

Since the late 1990s, statutory responsibility for 'social care' and specifically 'adult social care'[1] policy in the UK has been 'devolved' to the four national administrations, enabling England, Scotland, Wales and Northern Ireland to introduce their own legislation and standards, and allocate funding according to their own priorities (Gray and Birrell, 2013). This chapter focuses specifically on England, where the delivery of publicly funded adult social care services is the responsibility of 152 local authorities. The guiding principles shaping social care legislation and policy in England are currently 'prevention', 'person-centred care' and 'well-being' (Hall et al, 2020), all enshrined in the Care Act 2014 (see Box 2.1 for key statistics on adult social care expenditure, unmet need and the contribution of unpaid carers).

English local authorities receive an annual overall service budget from central government from which they part-fund adult social care, in addition to other sources of funding:

- each local authorities' own central budget, which includes revenue from business rates, charges to users of adult social care services and a 'social care precept' (that is, revenue from council tax since 2015);
- the National Health Service (NHS) budget;
- other central government sources, including extra money to ease 'winter pressures' on the NHS and the Social Care Support Grant (which covers adult social care and children's services).

BOX 2.1: SOCIAL CARE IN ENGLAND: KEY STATISTICS

- Total public expenditure by local authorities on adult social care in 2019–20 was £16.5 billion (NAO, 2021).
- The value of self-funded care was estimated to amount to £8.3 billion a year (NAO, 2021), though robust data on this market is lacking.
- The value of unpaid care was estimated to amount to more than £100 billion a year provided by 7.3 million carers in England (pre-COVID-19) (NAO, 2021).
- It is estimated that 24 per cent of those over the age of 65 in England had an unmet care need in 2018 (most recent available data; NAO, 2021).
- Around 1.5 million people in England worked in social care in 2019–20 (NAO, 2021).
- 97 per cent of local authority-funded home care is provided by the independent sector, including not-for-profit and for-profit companies (Homecare Association, 2021).
- In 2019–20, 839,000 people received adult social care arranged by local authorities (NAO, 2021).

Following the 2008 global financial crisis, a Conservative-led coalition government introduced a policy of austerity, the impact of which was keenly felt in adult social care in England. After taking transfers of funding from the NHS budget (7.5 per cent of public spending on social care in 2015–16) into account, over a six-year period (2009/10–2015/16), total local authority spending on all types of social care fell by 8.4 per cent, and by 16.8 per cent on adult social care specifically (Luchinskaya et al, 2017). However, individual local authority data show that cuts to spending on social care services were uneven. About one in seven local authorities increased such spending, while over the same six years, one in ten made cuts of more than 25 per cent (Phillips and Simpson, 2017). Local authorities that cut their social care spending hardest were in London boroughs (where cuts averaged 18 per cent) and in the metropolitan districts (16 per cent), including Greater Manchester, Tyneside and Greater Birmingham (Phillips and Simpson, 2017). The cuts were also unevenly experienced by different groups of people using adult social care, with older users of adult social care services experiencing greater reduction of provision than younger age groups (Glasby et al, 2020).

Eligibility for adult social care in England is both needs- and means-tested. 'National Care and Support (Eligibility Criteria) Regulations', set out in 2015 to guide implementation of the Care Act 2014, state that needs are eligible if a person meets specified criteria related to impairment, illness and lack of capacity to look after themselves that negatively affect their well-being. Until 2025, if a person in need of support has capital assets above £23,250, they must fund their own adult social care; those with £14,250–23,250 must contribute £1 per week for every £250 of savings they have; and those with less than £14,250 receive fully funded care. 'Capital assets' for people receiving a home or community care service are limited to savings only; for people in residential care facilities, such as care homes, this is based on their savings and the market value of their home. In 2021, changes were introduced to come into force in 2023 and then delayed until 2025 in November 2022, including a lifetime cap on the costs of personal care of £86,000 (excluding accommodation and 'hotel costs') and changes to the capital asset limits, with those with over £100,000 paying for their own care; those with between £20,000 and £100,000 contributing to the costs of their care; and those with less than £20,000 in assets receiving free state-provided care. State-provided adult social care can either be delivered by local authorities directly or through commissioned services, or the person can opt to receive a direct payment, which they can use to organise and fund their own care (although what they intend to spend their payments on requires local authority approval).

Given this rather tight 'rationing' of access to publicly funded support, it is unsurprising that, as in many other countries, the majority of all care provided to adults with care and support needs is provided by unpaid carers, typically family members, neighbours or friends. Under the Care Act 2014, these unpaid carers also have a right to have their own needs (and means) assessed, with support provided subject to meeting similar eligibility criteria.

Social care and technology: policy and practice in England

Technology and care policy: funding, delivery, eligibility and key principles

For the last 20 years, policy makers in England have advocated technology as one way to alleviate the 'crisis' in adult social care and improve outcomes, with over 25 UK government and official reports promoting the use of technology in care published in 25 years (Barlow et al, 2012). More recently, technology featured as a core theme in the 2021 White Paper 'People at the Heart of Care', which proposed £150 million in funding to 'drive greater adoption of technology and achieve widespread digitisation' (DHSC, 2021: 7).

Costs are an important rationale in the use of technology in social care in England, with many directors of adult social care seeing technology as crucial for containing budgets; 92 per cent of adult social care directors agreed that using 'assistive and communications technology' was 'quite' or 'very' important in making savings (ADASS, 2021). Local authority technology provision is largely funded from their local authority adult social care budgets, although some dedicated national funding streams have been made available (Wright, 2020). The impetus and funding to develop telecare and telehealth services in England over the past 20 or so years have come from a variety of central government sources, including departments responsible for health and social care, housing, and technology/digital investments, and from private industry. Central funding for research and development of new technologies has come mainly from national research bodies, including Innovate UK (formerly the Technology Strategy Board [TSB]), the National Institute for Health and Care Research (NIHR), UK Research and Innovation (UKRI) and NHS England, as well as from European Union research programmes. Examples of these funding opportunities are explored later in this chapter. Most decisions about piloting or implementing specific technologies have been taken by local authorities, in line with their statutory adult social care responsibilities, but the introduction of 'Integrated Care Systems' in 2022 may see joint endeavours between social care and the NHS provision locally. This combination of a mainly 'top-down' approach to research and development in technology and a more 'bottom-up' approach to budget allocation and implementation at the local level has led to a problematic 'disconnect', contributing to asymmetries in funding, knowledge and expertise, and a lack of participation in the design of new technologies by intended users. As Hendy et al put it (2012: 1), 'The implementation of a complex innovation such as remote care requires it to organically evolve, be responsive and adaptable to the local health and social care system, driven by support from front-line staff and management'.

Delivery of technology within adult social care varies between local authorities, but devices and associated services, including assessment, installation, monitoring and response, are increasingly 'contracted out'. Commissioning cycles for services vary, with some local authorities tied into long-term contracts with external organisations. Charging and assessment policies are also diverse, but again increasingly, local authorities no longer provide free technology services. Response arrangements for local authority-provided services also differ, with some offering a dedicated service while others require users to designate geographically close friends, neighbours or relatives to this role, or automatically contact the emergency services. Many local authorities are members of the 'Technology Enabled Care Services Association' (TSA), the main industry body for telecare and telehealth in England (and the UK), whose role includes lobbying government on issues related to technology in care. The TSA maintains a close relationship with local authority adult social care directors, who (via their own association, the Association of Directors of Adult Social Services [ADASS]) have been strong advocates of digital technology and see it as a key way to manage care workforce shortages (ADASS, 2019).

Use of technologies in social care practice

Telecare and telehealth

'Telecare' refers to a suite of diverse technologies aimed at enabling (mainly older) people to live for as long as possible in their own homes by connecting them with care services, while 'telehealth' refers to the remote monitoring of people with long-term conditions to enable a greater degree of self-management. Typically, telecare devices send an alert to someone outside of the property, generally an 'Alarm Receiving Centre' (ARC) who then either determines it is a false alert or summons additional help to the property (from named responders, a dedicated response service or the emergency services). Policy documents have referred to Doughty et al's (1996) 'three generations' model of telecare: the first comprises relatively cheap, reliable personal response and alarm services, enabling a user to indicate an emergency (for example, user-worn pendant alarms); the second, continuous smart sensors and monitoring using algorithms to raise an alarm autonomously if an emergency is detected (for example, fall detectors; gas carbon monoxide, temperature extreme sensors; bed and door exit sensors); and the third predicted the use of devices such as teleconferencing to create a 'virtual neighbourhood' to combat loneliness or forgetfulness and provide personal care, as well as complex sensors that can diagnose medical conditions, predict falls or remind users to take medication.

In practice, elements of all three generations of telecare co-exist and telecare and telehealth, under the overarching label 'Technology Enabled Care Services' (TECS), have become an increasingly core, albeit locally highly variable and unevenly distributed, component of England's adult social care technology landscape. The proliferation of telecare seems to have been a key means by which local authorities have maintained service provision, despite the aforementioned reductions to their budgets in recent years, and is also linked to the 'ageing in place' agenda, shifting the location of care away from expensive residential services. Technology in this context is used to manage risks, particularly for those living alone in later life or upon discharge from hospital.

First generation telecare devices have been part of social care arrangements since the 1960s in the form of simple community alarms: pull cords or buttons in homes to call for help in an emergency (Doughty et al, 1996). UK governments first made major investments in telecare projects in the late 1990s, following the inclusion of telecare in a White Paper on information strategy, part of an initiative to develop 'wired communities' (NHS Executive – Department of Health, 1998, cited in Akdur, 2019). By 2005, approximately 1.4 million people in England were being supported using community alarm service infrastructure (DH, 2005). A large-scale upgrading of telecare subsequently took place with national government investment in a two-year, £80 million Preventative Technology Grant. Total public expenditure on telecare in England in 2006–8 was £132 million, leading to rapid growth in the user base, with almost 150,000 new telecare users in 2006/7 and a further 161,000 in 2007/8 (Joint Improvement Team, 2008). Sources of additional funding for telecare later came to include a Better Care Fund allocation, local investments made by NHS clinical commissioning groups, and income from the fees paid by some telecare users (Woolham et al, 2018). The UK government's active promotion of telecare, primarily through the Preventative Technology Grant, was recognised by the European Commission in 2010 as 'probably the most comprehensive example internationally to date' (European Commission, 2010: iv), putting the UK into a leadership position in Europe in terms of disseminating this technology.

This policy investment in telecare services was followed by increased resources to develop an evidence base to promote uptake. The Department of Health launched a £31 million 'Whole System Demonstrator' (WSD) programme in 2008, aiming to conduct a robust randomised controlled trial to improve understanding of the impact of integrated telehealth and telecare. The largest such trial of telecare and telehealth services in the world, the WSD explored their cost, clinical effectiveness, patient and carer quality of life, and the everyday practices of health and social care professionals (DH, 2011; see section on 'Recent research evidence' below). The WSD included participants with chronic obstructive pulmonary disease, coronary heart disease and diabetes, as well as people with social care needs (with people with dementia specifically excluded).

The Department of Health launched a second major telecare and telehealth project in 2011, 3millionlives (3ML), in an £18 million investment over four years by the TSB (DH, 2012). 3ML aimed to 'scale up' the use of these services by developing the market, improving the global competitiveness of the UK telecare and telehealth industry, and improving users' quality of life through self-management at home. The TSB was also involved in several subsequent projects, including a £46 million investment via the Innovate Assisted Living Innovation Platform programmes (2011–13), designed to investigate how 'inexpensive, commodity-based services and devices could support older people'. In 2012, it launched a three-year project 'Delivering Assisted Living Lifestyles at Scale' (Dallas), aiming to build on the WSD and 3ML and 'to transform digitally supported self-care'. Dallas focused on improving knowledge about and access to existing services, rather than providing new services. It was supported by £19 million from the TSB, £1 million from NIHR, and £5 million from the Scottish government and from Highlands and Islands Enterprise and Scottish Enterprise (DH, 2016).

A further five-year £1.8 million randomised controlled trial, ATTILA (Assistive Technology and Telecare to maintain Independent Living At home for people with dementia), was launched in 2013. Reflecting an intensifying focus over the past decade on people living with dementia, this involved a collaboration between NIHR, NHS Foundation Trusts and local authorities, and aimed to evaluate whether telecare could safely extend the period people living with dementia could live independently in their own homes, and to what extent this would be cost-effective (see section on 'Recent research evidence' below).

Digital technology beyond telecare

Care technology in England has long been synonymous with telecare. However, this began to change in the 2010s, with a broader range of digital information and communications technology (ICT) devices entering the care landscape. While the market continues to be dominated by large telecare equipment providers such as Tunstall Healthcare and Legrand, new entrants have also emerged. Some essentially provide an extension of the capabilities of 'traditional' telecare, offering multifunctional devices that can be used to provide 'care at a distance' in the user's own home or, increasingly, outside in the community, to maintain their 'independence', while also gathering data that can be aggregated and used to manage care or predict future needs. There has also been a proliferation of medical devices and apps for consumer use at home. Some of these technologies target a younger demographic than their more established competitors, aiming to give reassurance to users and their families to provide more preventive data tracking services, and integrating new monitoring and analytics functionality with existing wearable consumer devices not specifically aimed at the care market (Wright, 2019).

In the 2010s, significant funding resources were utilised for research and development of ICT and robotics for care. The European Commission was a major funder, spending at least €235 million, composed of a mixture of public and private funding, across its Seventh and Eighth Framework Programmes for Research and Innovation between 2007 and 2020 (Wright, 2021a). English organisations participated in many of these European projects and some were 'part-hosted' at major robotics research centres in England (for example, Bristol Robotics Laboratory, Sheffield Robotics, and the universities of Hertfordshire, Bedfordshire and Plymouth). Examples include the €4.8 million 2011–2014 ambient assisted living (AAL) project Accompany, involving the trial of the Fraunhofer Institute's Care-O-Bot 3 at the University of Hertfordshire's Robot House, a smart home environment designed to test robots to 'support independent living in later life'. In 2017–20, €2.1 million of Horizon 2020 funding was spent on the Caresses project, hosted at the University of Bedfordshire, which aims to develop 'culturally competent' assistive social robots. The European Commission has also awarded funding to projects focused on ICT in social care more broadly, under the Seventh Framework Programme topic 'ICT and Ageing', and co-financed Pre-Commercial Procurement or Public Procurement of Innovative Solutions – programmes to encourage the private sector to develop commercial ICT care solutions (Wright, 2020).

Other key UK funding bodies for the research and development of ICT and robotics for care include Innovate UK and UKRI, which includes the Engineering and Physical Sciences Research Council (EPSRC). Major projects in the 2010s included the 'Trustworthy Robotic Assistants' programme at Bristol Robotics Laboratory (£1.2 million, 2013–16), funded by EPSRC, which aimed to investigate how robotic assistants can be used safely at home. Designability's CHIRON assistive robotic systems to enable older people to live at home for longer received £2.2 million in 2016–18 from Innovate UK (DH, 2017). CHIRON was a collaboration between Bristol City Council, Bristol Robotics Laboratory and Designability, and tested the 'Pepper' and 'Nao' robots. Despite the promise of such research projects, and significant investment by governments, the utility and cost-effectiveness of many of these robotic prototypes remain unproven; very few have been commercialised or are widely available. Those products that have been commercialised are often extremely expensive; for example, the humanoid robot Pepper cost around US$25,000 leased over a period of three years before production was discontinued in 2021, and Paro, a seal-shaped therapy robot, cost £5,000 excluding taxes at time of writing. Local authorities have tended to rely on collaborations with academic researchers to trial care robots and other emerging technologies. An exception is the Argenti partnership's piloting of the exoskeleton HAL, produced by the Japanese company Cyberdyne, in collaboration with Hampshire Council, funded by a Local Government Association (LGA) grant (Wright, 2020).

Robotics research projects typically take years to translate into consumer products that can be used safely, effectively and affordably in homes or care facilities – if at all. However, in the past five years, widely available, relatively cheap consumer electronics, including tablets, smartphones, virtual assistants and apps, have been trialled for use in local authority adult social care. One factor driving local authority interest in this area is the significant challenge facing the 'traditional' first and second generation TECS sector due to the 2025 digital switchover, which will render devices that rely on analogue telephone lines unreliable or unusable (Hamblin, 2020). It is estimated that the replacement of analogue devices with digital equivalents will cost UK local authorities £150–300 million (TSA, 2017), and it is unclear if local authorities are adequately prepared for this switchover despite government departments and organisations, such as the TSA (2017), repeatedly highlighting the issue. At the same time, there has been a boom in the use of 'smart' home systems (that is, networked sets of home sensors, appliances and heating/cooling under digital control) and personal consumer digital devices (for example, smart watches, voice-controlled virtual assistants, such as Amazon's Alexa, and wearable fitness monitoring devices, such as Fitbit and Apple Watch). The 2021 government White Paper (DHSC, 2021) includes examples of how mainstream 'smart' devices are being used in social care arrangements. Though such devices, such as Amazon's voice-controlled virtual assistant Alexa, were not specifically designed for use in care settings and generally have not yet been integrated into existing TECS systems, they have been tested by several local authorities, including Oxfordshire, Norfolk, Richmond and Hampshire, with special Alexa functions or 'skills' to remind users to take medication and to record and manage care tasks completed by both paid care workers and unpaid carers (Wright, 2021b; Hamblin, 2022a, b). Trials of these kinds of consumer devices have been encouraged by the Care and Health Improvement Programme (CHIP), introduced in 2014/15 by the LGA in partnership with ADASS and NHS England. CHIP's Social Care Digital Innovation Programme has been a major driver for local authorities' experimentation with different technologies and has provided numerous small grants to fund pilot projects.

Self-service websites offering online information about social care services and health and self-care advice were also an important area of development in the 2010s. A 2012 government White Paper ('Caring for our future: reforming care and support'; HM Government, 2012) promised £32.5 million in start-up funding over two years from 2014 to 2015 for local authorities to develop websites providing information about local care and support (De Leonibus et al,

2013), and the 2021 White Paper proposed a national website offering information about adult social care reform, as well as £5 million to 'pilot new ways to help people understand and access the care and support available' (DHSC, 2021: 8). Part of this focus on websites involved the development of new online assessment tools.

Software apps for mobile phones and tablets also gained prominence as a technology that can be relatively quick and inexpensive to develop, makes use of existing hardware infrastructure, is readily scalable and is relatively interoperable across different consumer devices (De Leonibus et al, 2013). ADASS again took a leading role in encouraging their development. In 2015, it organised an 'ADASS Care Apps Showcase' featuring presentations from developers about apps to support social care, and set up an online showcase, 'Public Service Digital eXchange', to bring together adult social care commissioners and app developers. Modest funding was also provided by Innovate UK, among other funders. Increasingly, companies – such as Supercarers, Elder, My Home Touch and TrustonTap – have developed apps and platforms that connect care workers with people who need support.

ICT infrastructure and data

Many of the emergent care technologies described above are premised on users having reliable broadband connections at home to access and use the Internet. While 92 per cent of adults in the UK had used the Internet in the previous three months, this figure dropped to 54 per cent of those over the age of 75 in 2020 (ONS, 2020). Internet access and use are therefore a significant obstacle affecting the aim to provide Internet-based digital services in older adults' homes to support independence (Hamblin, 2022a).

The speed of Internet and data connections also depend on geographically contingent technological infrastructure. Ofcom, the UK's communications regulator, reported that in 2020 in England, around 119,000 homes and businesses could not receive broadband speeds of at least 10 Mbit/s download and 1 Mbit/s upload over a fixed line or fixed wireless connection, and of these, 54 per cent were in rural areas; average download speeds were also significantly lower in rural areas (52 Mbit/s compared to 78 Mbit/s in urban areas) (Ofcom, 2020). The 2021 social care White Paper acknowledged these issues and proposed working with telecommunications providers to improve connectivity to ensure home care providers and residential care settings could 'work digitally' (DHSC, 2021: 44) to enhance work underway from 2020 to create a Shared Rural Network (a collaboration between government and the UK's four mobile network operators to deliver 4G coverage to 95 per cent of the UK) (Ofcom, 2020).

Integration of social care with health (and housing and other public services) continues to be on the policy agenda in England. Many government departments and independent agencies see ICT as crucial in reaching this goal. Meanwhile, low levels of information sharing and digital interoperability, and new information governance structures are seen as barriers to integration (CQC, 2018; Booth-Smith, 2017; LGA, 2013). NHS Foundation Trusts often use different systems, making it difficult to digitalise and share NHS electronic patient records, and many local adult social care systems have resorted to resource-intensive workarounds (LGA, 2013). The complexity of this task has intensified as numbers of telecare and telehealth devices, monitoring systems and care management systems have proliferated, each generating their own sets of user data. Attempts have been made to improve integration, for example, through the Dallas project's 2012–15 i-Focus initiative. In 2015, NHS England set out a 'Five Year Forward View' and a 'Personalised Health and Care 2020' plan for using ICT and ensuring patient records are digitised and interoperable by 2020 (NHS England et al, 2014). The Health and Social Care (Safety and Quality) Act 2015 reinforced the pressure for integration, making it a legal requirement to share information where it is likely to facilitate the provision of health or care services and is in the individual's 'best interests'.

An important goal of integration is to enable patient records and other data to be aggregated in one place. Yet the growth of historic and real-time data on individuals and their care available to local authorities has created new technical issues relating to data governance and organisational culture and raises significant ethical questions about how personal data should be protected or used, by whom and for what purpose. Many local authorities lack the resources or technical capacity to use the huge amounts of data generated by the boom in telecare since the mid-2000s (ADASS, 2019). Nationally, a Health and Social Care Information Centre was established in 2013 (rebranded 'NHS Digital' in 2016), with a remit to include health and social care services. At the local level, however, specific expertise in data science is often lacking, and organisational culture may not be conducive to using data (CQC, 2018). Again, this was highlighted as an area of focus in the 2021 White Paper, with the proposed creation of an 'adult social care data framework' and new requirements for data collection placed on local authorities (DHSC, 2021).

Several local authority data analytics projects and pilots have focused on care prevention. Shropshire Council's 'The Bridge' project (part-funded by CHIP's Social Care Digital Innovation Programme) combined datasets from the NHS, adult social care and the Office for National Statistics, as well as thermal mapping of homes, aiming to improve the efficiency of commissioning and enable preventive care by identifying 'those in a cold home, over 75, living alone and not known to social care' (SCIE, 2018; LGA and NHS Digital, 2019). Other preventive projects include ARMED, developed by HAS Technology, which uses various in-home sensors and a wearable device to gather physiological data to predict the risk of falling and intervene to prevent this; a 2018–2020 trial indicated that this produced data that could predict falls with a high degree of accuracy (Digital Health Wales, 2020).

Other local authorities have turned to technology and artificial intelligence (AI) companies for data analytics and insight, reflecting a broader shift towards state investment in and focus on AI as part of the UK government's Industrial Strategy. In August 2019, plans to create a national AI lab for the NHS in England were announced to manage 'the digitisation of the health and care service', within a broader £250 million investment. At the local level, Harrow Council utilised IBM's Watson Care Manager and several local authorities use Amazon's Alexa, linked to Amazon Web Services, which can store and analyse user data. However, the practice of providing technology corporations with access to citizens' personal data is coming under increasing scrutiny, especially since implementation of the European General Data Protection Regulation in 2018, legislated for in the UK in the *Data Protection Act 2018* which introduced new data protection and privacy rules governing citizens' data. The Department of Health also published a code of conduct for data-driven health and care technology in 2018 following criticism of Alphabet company DeepMind and the NHS by the Information Commissioner's Office for failure to comply with the Data Protection Act in using NHS patient data. Despite this, highly problematic data governance practices persist (Walker, 2019).

Impact of the COVID-19 pandemic

The COVID-19 pandemic in many ways advanced the use of technologies in adult social care, in particular mainstream devices. At the national level, the process of allowing care providers free access to NHSmail – an email, diary and directory system for NHS employees in England and Scotland – was accelerated and information governance compliance requirements were relaxed to promote information flows between health and social care (IPC, 2020). At the local authority level, a variety of different approaches were undertaken, such as using Amazon Web Services' automated 'robocall' service, mainstream devices such as smart speakers (for example, Hampshire County Council) or Microsoft 'Power Apps' (Bury Council), to contact and check the well-being of residents on the 'shielding' lists (TSA, 2021). Mainstream devices were also provided nationally, with the former Secretary of State for Health and Social Care, Matt Hancock, announcing 11,000 iPads would be made available to avoid 'unnecessary' in-person visits to care homes (Wright, 2021b), and locally, with local authorities using similar devices (for example, North Yorkshire County Council, Staffordshire County Council and Stoke-on-Trent Council; IPC et al, 2020). There were also examples of local authorities working to ensure these mainstream devices could be used through the provision of support to develop digital skills (for example, Stockport Metropolitan Borough Council and DigiKnow; IPC et al, 2020).

Recent research evidence on the use of technology in English social care

There is significant debate about the quality and type of evidence required in the research of technology in adult social care, particularly between proponents of randomised controlled trials (Davies and Newman, 2011) and those who argue that technologies deployed in social care are 'complex interventions' that cannot be evaluated in isolation from their contexts (Hamblin et al, 2017; Eccles, 2020). Williams et al (2003: 52) argue questions about the effectiveness of telecare are a matter of politics between disciplines in a multidisciplinary field characterised by 'significant contests and disagreements not only over the kinds of evidence that are persuasive of effectiveness, but also by territorial disputes about whose knowledge is authoritative'.

In England, early qualitative studies of telecare have found that telecare provided a sense of security for users (Horton, 2008) and supports 'ageing in place' (Poole, 2006), but that important contextual factors mediate its experience and use (Hamblin et al, 2017) and its deployment may have unintended consequences, including the confinement of users to their home environment (Aceros et al, 2015; Lariviere et al, 2021). Those who stress the importance of context argue that telecare 'might best be summarised as applicable to some people, in some circumstances, at some points in their lives. In short, it has been less of a panacea than policy agendas initially suggested' (Eccles, 2020: 3). At the local authority level, commissioned telecare services in England have been critiqued for neglecting users' aspirations, well-being and desired outcomes (Lynch et al, 2019).

Qualitative studies have also explored the impact of telecare on unpaid carers, finding services can treat them as a 'resource' (Steils et al, 2021) but also that it took 'a weight off my mind' (Jarrold and Yeandle, 2009). Research including care workers indicated their ambivalence toward telecare (Yeandle and Fry, 2010) and its limited impact on job roles (Hanson et al, 2007), while other earlier studies have found them to be extremely positive about the benefits of telecare for the people they support and their families (Magnusson et al, 2005), their ability to carry out their role effectively and the opportunities for professional skill development they felt it could offer (Alaszewski and Cappello, 2006). Research has also examined the roles technology in care provision creates, in alarm receiving centres or as emergency responders, suggesting that although they are integral to 'co-producing' ageing in place and care (Wigfield et al, 2012; Wigfield et al, 2013; Procter et al, 2014), they are seen as conducting 'data work' (Grisot et al, 2019) and there are implications for esteem and job quality (Roberts et al, 2012; Hamblin, 2022b).

In response to the demand for 'robust evidence', the aforementioned WSD was developed to provide an evidence base beyond small-scale, qualitative and device-specific projects. The WSD pointed to significant benefits from tele*health*, but the tele*care* aspect of the trial did not demonstrate similar gains in any of the sixteen measured outcomes (Steventon et al, 2013). The telecare strand of the WSD indicated 'no statistically significant' differences between the intervention and control groups in terms of admissions to residential care or to hospital (Steventon et al, 2013) and no demonstrable cost savings (Henderson et al, 2014). Telecare users' (and their carers') quality of life, measured in terms of mental health and anxiety, while 'enhanced' were not 'transformed' (Hirani et al, 2014). Nonetheless, Eccles (2020) highlights that these findings did not dampen the government's enthusiasm for telecare, noting that the Dallas research programme was launched to provide the missing evidence on cost savings, but reported *after* the 3ML programme had already been funded. As such, he observes 'policy makers were still on the same trajectory of ignoring the inconvenience of evidence' (Eccles, 2020: 13). The approach of English governments to telecare policy and its evidence base has therefore been critiqued (Eccles, 2020) for 'implementing telecare technologies on a large scale and on a top-down basis [which is] a hazardous investment' (Pols and Willems, 2011: 496).

Woolham et al (2018) argue the findings of the WSD presented significant problems for the government and many local authorities that were heavily invested, financially and politically, in telecare, as well as for telecare manufacturers and suppliers. Perhaps as a result of this, the WSD findings have had little bearing on local authorities' commissioning approaches to TECS (Woolham et al, 2018). There were also critiques regarding the presentation of the WSD's findings, accusations of 'cherry picking' (Greenhalgh, 2012) and negative comments on its methodology. Other research has acknowledged shortcomings in the WSD trial but concluded that its results were not necessarily 'wrong' – a view nevertheless widespread among local authorities (Woolham et al, 2018). The aforementioned ATTILA trial's results also found limited positive effects, reporting telecare did not increase the length of time that participants with dementia lived outside of residential care settings and did not decrease caregiver 'burden', depression or anxiety, with carers often responsible for managing technology (Gathercole et al, 2021; Lariviere et al, 2021).

Use of new digital technologies in adult social care has tended to be based on small trials, leading some to use the term 'pilot fatigue' or 'pilot-itis' (Barlow and Hendy, 2009; Barlow et al, 2012) to refer to the lack of delivery at scale in relation to their application (Hamblin, 2020). The evidence base for many new technological devices is underdeveloped, an issue exacerbated by the continuous proliferation of devices and the shorter lifecycles of many generic consumer products that local authorities are introducing into care, making their inclusion in rigorous, long-term peer-reviewed studies difficult. There have been recent signs of a change of approach: 'NHSX' was set up in July 2019 to bring teams from the Department of Health and Social Care, NHS England and NHS Improvement together to 'drive digital transformation and lead policy, implementation and change', while Digital Social Care (a group of organisations including provider organisations, working with NHS Digital) was established in the same year to 'provide advice and support to the sector on technology and data protection'. More recently, NHS Digital, NHSX, NHS Improvement and NHS England have been merged into a single organisation: the NHS Transformation Directorate. In the area of medical apps, ORCHA assesses quality and efficacy for NHS organisations, and NHSX launched the Digital Technology Assessment Criteria in 2021 to establish a common baseline standard for apps and other digital health technologies. However, at time of writing, equivalent standards and tools to assess social care applications of emerging technologies not directly related to health had not yet been established. The 2021 White Paper includes the aim that people using care services should 'have confidence in selecting and using the most appropriate digital tools to support their independence, safety, and wellbeing, knowing which technologies meet essential standards' (DHSC,

2021: 42) and refers to 'proven technologies', but with no detail on who will lead or implement these standards. There are debates around the security of mainstream 'smart' and 'Internet of things' devices, with the 2022 'Product Security and Telecoms Infrastructure Bill' striving to create requirements for manufacturers and sellers of these devices to ensure they are less vulnerable to cyber-attacks. However, at the time of writing in autumn 2022, it is the voluntary 2018 Code of Practice for Consumer IoT Security that applies to many technologies currently being trialled in adult social care.

Conclusion

Throughout the 2010s, England's social care system was widely characterised as 'broken', a situation reinforced by major real-terms cuts to local authority budgets. The system has become ever more precarious, with multiple care home and home care companies in administration or close to collapse, a precarious workforce with a high attrition rate and very low pay, and some older people having to use most of their assets to fund their care. A lack of political leadership in addressing problems of funding, delivery and the workforce in adult social care has meant some local authorities have come to see technology, with the opportunities and risks it brings, as a main focus of their strategic planning.

The digital transformation underway in adult social care and the NHS, as in the wider economy, is also creating compelling opportunities for data collection and sharing to drive improved outcomes for older people. Many policy documents and reports nevertheless identify high cost, the digital divide with deficiencies of digital access, literacy and infrastructure, lack of interoperability between new and legacy systems, and data governance challenges (including privacy and data security) as barriers to the wider adoption of new technologies (Booth-Smith, 2017; CQC, 2018; Hamblin, 2020). Care users with direct payments or personal budgets may consider using these to purchase assistive devices, but have low awareness of available technologies and what they can do, while the marketplace in which they can be purchased remains highly fragmented (De Leonibus et al, 2013).

At the close of the 2010s, this fragmentation reflected a lack of national-level funding or strategic ambition to promote new technologies, in contrast to the substantial funding available for widespread implementation of telecare in the early 2000s. In effect, implementation of much new technology for social care has been left to local authorities, which have limited technical capacities, capabilities and resources to assess emerging technologies and make informed and effective commissioning decisions. This has created bottlenecks that impede their effective use, while trials of relatively expensive new technologies such as robotics have remained small-scale and inconclusive about benefits and cost savings.

A further problem is that a local authority-based approach to the adoption and implementation of sophisticated new technologies may contribute to already worrying inequalities in distribution. Local authorities have varying levels of expertise in specialised areas like data science and AI, and the procurement skills needed to win innovation funding and use it effectively or to bring together and manage complex public–private consortia (such as the PA Argenti partnership model deployed in Hampshire and Barnet). This is creating a fundamental mismatch between local authorities' responsibility for delivering social care at the local level, which can lead to the emergence of 'local silos', and the growing need to plan and implement interoperable and highly complex systems across the country to gather, analyse and action big data sets in real time.

The COVID-19 pandemic has accelerated technology use in adult social care, but again, with considerable local variations and inequalities. The 2021 White Paper's (DHSC, 2021) focus on technology includes reference to a 'social care technology blueprint' that could contribute to a national strategy in England, rather than multiple local initiatives, and thereby facilitate the successful scale and spread of effective technology use in adult social care. While far from a magic bullet that will 'fix' England's social care system, the potential for new and emerging technologies to improve the quality of care remains largely untapped, and considerable vision and leadership, careful planning and research, and robust governance mechanisms will be required to deliver its benefits in a safe, secure and sustainable manner.

Note

1 In 2005, 'adult social care' was separated from services for children due to concerns over the quality of provision for the latter (Hall et al, 2020).

References

Aceros, J.C., Pols, J. and Domènech, M. (2015) 'Where is grandma? Home telecare, good aging and the domestication of later life', *Technological Forecasting and Social Change*, 93: 102–111.

Akdur, G. (2019) 'Redefining the identity of old age through telecare: A Foucauldian inquiry into national care policies and practices at local social care authorities', PhD thesis, Department of Management, Information Systems and Innovation Group, London School of Economics and Political Science.

Alaszewski, A. and Cappello, R. (2006) 'Piloting telecare in Kent County Council: the key lessons – final report'. Canterbury: Kent County Council and University of Kent.

Association of Directors of Adult Social Services [ADASS]. (2019) 'Connected social care: Adult social care leaders explore the pros, cons and challenges of tech-enabled care', New Dialogues Report Spring 2019. Available at: https://www.adass.org.uk/media/6804/tunstall-round-table-connected-social-care.pdf [accessed 18.01.23].

Association of Directors of Adult Social Services. (2021) 'ADASS Budget Survey 2019: ADASS Spring Survey 2021'. Available at: https://www.adass.org.uk/adass-spring-survey-21 [accessed 10.02.2022].

Barlow, J. and Hendy, J. (2009) 'Adopting integrated mainstream telecare services', *Chronic Disease Management and Remote Patient Monitoring,* 15(1): 8.

Barlow, J., Hendy, J. and Chrysanthaki, T. (2012) 'Scaling-up remote care in the united kingdom: lessons from a decade of policy intervention', in Glascock, A. and Kutzik, D. (Eds) *Essential Lessons for the Success of Telehomecare – Why It's not Plug and Play*, Amsterdam: IOS Press.

Booth-Smith, L. (2017) 'Rebooting health and social care integration: an agenda for more person centred care', London: Localis. Available at: https://www.localis.org.uk/wp-content/uploads/2017/07/HASC-report-final.pdf [accessed 21.02.23].

Care Quality Commission [CQC]. (2018) 'Beyond barriers: how older people move between health and social care in England', London: CQC. Available at: https://www.cqc.org.uk/publications/themed-work/beyond-barriers-how-older-people-move-between-health-care-england [accessed 21.02.23].

Davies, A. and Newman, S. (2011) 'Evaluating telecare and telehealth interventions', WSDAN briefing paper, London: Kings Fund.

De Leonibus, V., Bartosova, R. and Lewis, E. (2013) 'ALT market in the UK –AKTIVE market report: initial overview', AKTIVE research report, CIRCLE, Leeds: University of Leeds.

Department of Health [DH]. (2005) 'Building telecare in England', London: DH.

Department of Health. (2011) 'Research and development work relating to assistive technology 2010–11', London: DHSC. Available at: https://www.gov.uk/government/publications/research-and-development-work-relating-to-assistive-technology-2010-11 [accessed 21.02.23].

Department of Health. (2012) 'Caring for our future: reforming care and support', London: DH. Available at: https://www.gov.uk/government/publications/caring-for-our-future-reforming-care-and-support [accessed 21.02.23].

Department of Health. (2016) 'Research and development work relating to assistive technology 2015–16', London: DHSC. Available at: https://assets.publishing.service.gov.uk/government/uploads/system/uploads/attachment_data/file/553803/AT_RD_report_2015_16.pdf [accessed 21.02.23].

Department of Health. (2017) 'Research and development work relating to assistive technology 2016–17', London: DH. Available at: https://assets.publishing.service.gov.uk/government/uploads/system/uploads/attachment_data/file/775870/Research_and_development_work_relating_to_assistive_technology_2016_to_2017.pdf [accessed 21.02.23].

Department of Health and Social Care [DHSC]. (2021) 'People at the heart of care: adult social care reform', London: DHSC. Available at: https://www.gov.uk/government/publications/people-at-the-heart-of-care-adult-social-care-reform-white-paper/people-at-the-heart-of-care-adult-social-care-reform [accessed 21.02.23].

Digital Health Wales. (2020) 'ARMED'. Available at: https://digitalhealth.wales/projects/armed [accessed 01.08.22].

Doughty, K., Cameron, K. and Garner, P. (1996) 'Three generations of telecare of the elderly', *Journal of Telemedicine and Telecare*, 2(2): 71–80.

Eccles, A. (2020) 'Remote care technologies, older people, and the social care crisis in the United Kingdom: a multiple streams approach to understanding the "silver bullet" of telecare policy', *Ageing and Society*, 41(8): 1726–1747.

European Commission. (2010) 'ICT and ageing: European study on users, markets and technologies', prepared by empirica and WRC on behalf of the European Commission, Directorate General for Information Society and Media, Brussels: EC.

Gathercole, R., Bradley, R., Harper, E., Davis, L., Pank, L., Lam, N., et al (2021) 'Assistive technology and telecare to maintain independent living at home for people with dementia: the ATTILA RCT', *NIHR Health Technology Assessment*, 19: 1–156.

Glasby, J., Zhang, Y., Bennett, M.R. and Hall, P. (2020) 'A lost decade? A renewed case for adult social care reform in England', *Journal of Social Policy*, 50(2): 406–437.

Gray, A. M. and Birrell, D. (2013) *Transforming Adult Social Care*, Bristol: Policy Press.

Greenhalgh, T. (2012) 'Whole System Demonstrator trial: policy, politics, and publication ethics', *British Medical Journal*, 345: e5280.

Grisot, M., Moltubakk Kempton, A., Hagen, L. and Aanestad, M. (2019) 'Data-work for personalized care: examining nurses' practices in remote monitoring of chronic patients', *Health Informatics Journal*, 25(3): 608–616.

Hall, P., Needham, C. and Hamblin, K. (2020) 'Social care', in Ellison, N. and Haux, T. (Eds) *Handbook of Society and Social Policy: Social Care*, Cheltenham: Edward Elgar, pp 321–332.

Hamblin, K. (2020) 'Technology and social care in a digital world: challenges and opportunities in the UK', *Journal of Enabling Technologies*, 14(2): 115–125.

Hamblin, K. (2022a) 'Sustainable social care: the potential of mainstream "smart" technologies', *Sustainability*, 14(5): 2754.

Hamblin, K. A. (2022b) 'Technology in care systems: displacing, reshaping, reinstating or degrading roles?' *New Technology, Work and Employment*, 37(1): 41–58.

Hamblin, K., Yeandle, S. and Fry, G. (2017) 'Researching telecare: the importance of context', *Journal of Enabling Technologies*, 11(3): 75–84.

Hanson, J., Percival, J., Aldred, H., Brownsell, S. and Hawley, M. (2007) 'Attitudes to telecare among older people, professional care workers and informal carers: a preventative strategy or crisis management?', *Univ Access Inf Soc*, 6: 193–205.

Henderson, C., Knapp, M., Fernández, J.L., Beecham, J., Hirani, S.P., Beynon, M., et al (2014) 'Cost-effectiveness of telecare for people with social care needs: the Whole Systems Demonstrator cluster randomised trial', *Age and Ageing*, 43(6): 794–800.

Hendy, J., Chrysanthaki, T., Barlow, J., Knapp, M., Rogers, A., Sanders, C., et al (2012) 'An organisational analysis of the implementation of telecare and telehealth: the whole systems demonstrator', *BMC Health Services Research*, 12(1): 1–10.

Hirani, S.P., Beynon, M., Cartwright, M., Rixon, L., Doll, H., Henderson, C., et al (2014) 'The effect of telecare on the quality of life and psychological well-being of elderly recipients of social care over a 12-month period: the Whole Systems Demonstrator cluster randomised trial', *Age and Ageing*, 43(3): 334–341.

HM Government. (2012) 'Caring for our future: reforming care and support', London: HMSO. Available at: https://www.gov.uk/government/publications/caring-for-our-future-reforming-care-and-support [accessed 21.02.23].

Homecare Association. (2021) 'An overview of the domiciliary care market in the UK'. Available at: https://www.homecareassociation.org.uk/resource/market-overview-2021.html [accessed 01.08.22].

Horton, K. (2008) 'Falls in older people: the place of telemonitoring in rehabilitation', *Journal of Rehabilitation Research and Development*, 45(8): 1183–1194.

IPC, ADASS and LGA. (2020) 'Digital innovation in adult social care: how we've been supporting communities during COVID-19 - executive summary', Oxford: IPC. Available at: https://www.local.gov.uk/publications/digital-innovation-adult-social-care-how-weve-been-supporting-communities-during-covid [accessed 21.02.23].

Jarrold, K. and Yeandle, S. (2009) 'A weight off my mind: exploring the impact and potential benefits of telecare for unpaid carers in Scotland', Glasgow: Carers Scotland.

Joint Improvement Team. (2008) 'Telecare in Scotland: benchmarking the present, embracing the future'. Joint Improvement Team Scotland.

Lariviere, M., Poland, F., Woolham, J., Newman, S. and Fox, C. (2021) 'Placing assistive technology and telecare in everyday practices of people with dementia and their caregivers: findings from an embedded ethnography of a national dementia trial', *BMC Geriatrics*, 21: 121.

Local Government Association [LGA]. (2013) 'Integrated care and support resource sheet', London: LGA. Available at: https://www.local.gov.uk/publications/integrated-care-and-support-resource-sheet [accessed 21.02.23].

Local Government Association and NHS Digital. (2019) 'Project Recap: redesign and empower the care provider market', Discovery review, London: LGA.

Luchinskaya, D., Simpson, P. and Stoye, G. (2017) 'UK health and social care spending' in Emmerson, C., Johnson, P. and Joyce, R. (Eds) *Institute for Fiscal Studies (IFS) Green Budget 2017*, London: Institute for Fiscal Studies, pp 141–176.

Lynch, J.K., Glasby, J. and Robinson, S. (2019) 'If telecare is the answer, what was the question? Storylines, tensions and the unintended consequences of technology-supported care', *Critical Social Policy*, 39(1): 44–65.

Magnusson, L., Hanson, E. and Nolan, M. (2005) 'The impact of information and communication technology on family carers of older people and professionals in Sweden', *Ageing and Society*, 25: 693–713.

National Audit Office [NAO]. (2021) 'The adult social care market in England'. Available at: https://www.nao.org.uk/report/adult-social-care-markets/ [accessed 01.08.22].

NHS England, CQC, Health Education England, Monitor, TDA and Public Health England. (2014) 'Five Year Forward View', London: NHS England. Available at: https://www.england.nhs.uk/wp-content/uploads/2014/10/5yfv-web.pdf [accessed 21.03.23].

NHS Executive – Department of Health. (1998) 'Information for health: an information strategy for the modern NHS 1998–2005'. London: Department of Health.

Ofcom. (2020) 'Connected Nations 2020'. Available at: https://www.ofcom.org.uk/research-and-data/multi-sector-research/infrastructure-research/connected-nations-2020 [accessed 28.06.22].

Office of National Statistics [ONS]. (2020) 'Internet users, UK: 2020'. Available at: https://www.ons.gov.uk/businessindustryandtrade/itandinternetindustry/bulletins/internetusers/2020 [accessed 28.06.22].

Phillips, D. and Simpson, P. (2017) 'National standards, local risks: the geography of local authority funded social care, 2009–10 to 2015–16', London: Institute for Fiscal Studies. Available at: https://ifs.org.uk/publications/national-standards-local-risks-geography-local-authority-funded-social-care-2009-10 [accessed 21.02.23].

Pols, J. and Willems, D. (2011) 'Innovation and evaluation: taming and unleashing telecare technology', *Sociology of Health and Illness*, 33(3): 484–498.

Poole, T. (2006) 'Wanless social care review: telecare and older people'. London: Kings Fund. Available at: https://www.kingsfund.org.uk/sites/files/kf/telecare-older-people-wanless-background-paper-teresa-poole2006.pdf [accessed 21.02.23].

Procter, R., Greenhalgh, T., Wherton, J., Sugarhood, P., Rouncefield, M. and Hinder, S. (2014) 'The day-to-day co-production of ageing in place', *Computer Supported Cooperative Work*, 23(3): 245–267.

Roberts, C., Mort, M. and Milligan, C. (2012) 'Calling for care: "disembodied" work, teleoperators and older people living at home', *Sociology*, 46(3): 490–506.

Social Care Institute for Excellence [SCIE]. (2018) 'Transforming Care and Support', London: SCIE.

Steils, N., Woolham, J., Fisk, M., Porteus, J. and Forsyth, K. (2021) 'Carers' involvement in telecare provision by local councils for older people in England: perspectives of council telecare managers and stakeholders', *Ageing and Society*, 41(2): 456–475.

Steventon, A., Bardsley, M., Billings, J., Dixon, J., Doll., H., Beynon, M., et al (2013) 'Effect of telecare on use of health and social care services: findings from the Whole Systems Demonstrator cluster randomised trial', *Age and Ageing*, 42(4): 501–508.

Technology Enabled Care Services Association [TSA]. (2017) 'Connecting people, improving lives: a digital future for Technology Enabled Care?' TSA White Paper, Wilmslow: TSA.

Technology Enabled Care Services Association. (2021) 'From stabilisation to innovation: the response and redesign of TEC services during COVID-19', Wilmslow: TSA.

Walker, A. (2019) 'NHS gives Amazon free use of health data under Alexa advice deal', *The Guardian*. Available at: https://www.theguardian.com/society/2019/dec/08/nhs-gives-amazon-free-use-of-health-data-under-alexa-advice-deal [accessed 18.01.23].

Wigfield, A., Moore, S., Buse, C. and Fry, G. (2012) 'Workforce development for assisted living technology: understanding roles, delivery and workforce needs', Leeds: CIRCLE. Available at: https://essl.leeds.ac.uk/download/downloads/id/307/circle_sept_final_doc1.pdf [accessed 21.02.23].

Wigfield, A., Wright, K., Burtney, E. and Buddery, D. (2013) 'Assisted living technology in social care: workforce development implications', *Journal of Assistive Technologies*, 7(4): 204–218.

Williams, T., May, C., Mair, F., Mort, M. and Gask, L. (2003) 'Normative models of health technology assessment and the social production of evidence about telehealth care', *Health Policy*, 64(1): 39–54.

Woolham, J. G., Steils, N., Fisk, M., Porteus, J. and Forsyth, K. (2018) 'The UTOPIA project: using telecare for older people in adult social care. The findings of a 2016–17 national survey of local authority telecare provision for older people in England', London: Social Care Workforce Research Unit, King's College London. Available at: https://kclpure.kcl.ac.uk/portal/en/publications/the-utopia-project-using-telecare-for-older-people-in-adult-social-care(fa425089-10a3-40ba-9eee-a96534bebc98)/export.html [accessed 21.02.23].

Wright, J. (2019) 'Robots vs migrants? Reconfiguring the future of Japanese institutional eldercare', *Critical Asian Studies*, 51(3): 331–354.

Wright, J. (2020) 'Technology in social care: review of the UK policy landscape', Centre for International Research on Care, Labour and Equalities. Available at: https://www.researchgate.net/publication/344954182_Technology_in_social_care_a_review_of_the_UK_policy_landscape [accessed 29.11.22].

Wright, J. (2021a) 'Comparing public funding approaches to the development and commercialization of care robots in the European Union and Japan', *Innovation: The European Journal of Social Science Research*, 1–16.

Wright, J. (2021b) 'The Alexafication of adult social care: virtual assistants and the changing role of local government in England', *International Journal of Environmental Research and Public Health*, 18(2): 812–824.

Yeandle, S. and Fry, G. (2010) 'The potential of ICT in supporting domiciliary care in England', Luxembourg: Publications Office of the European Union.

THREE

Technology to support ageing in place in Australia

Meryl Lovarini, Kate O'Loughlin and Lindy Clemson

Social care: policy, debates and evidence in Australia

Australia's aged care sector provides a range of services delivered in the home, in residential care facilities or as transitional and respite care to meet assessed needs (Department of Health, 2021a). All levels of government (national, state/territory, local) contribute to the sector; however, overall responsibility resides with the national government. Legislative and policy reforms in 2013 introduced a consumer-directed care (CDC) model as the framework to support older people's living and care arrangements, specifically focused on meeting their needs to remain in the community.

Levels of support pre- and post 2013

Prior to the reforms, two levels of support existed: low-intensity Home and Community Care Packages and high-intensity Community Age Care Packages. Government-approved for-profit or not-for-profit providers administered packages to community-dwelling clients. While this provided a guaranteed income for the provider, long waiting lists existed and incentives to respond to clients' needs were limited. A government-initiated investigation by the Productivity Commission (an organisation providing independent research and advice to the government on economic, social and environmental issues affecting the welfare of Australians) reported that extensive nationwide reforms were needed to overcome significant 'delays, discontinuities, constraints and shortages' (Productivity Commission, 2011: 19).

The Aged Care (Living Longer Living Better) Act 2013 introduced a CDC model to provide care and support for older Australians to 'age in place' (that is, to live outside of residential care settings). The reforms provided a market-based system to drive quality, innovation and sustainable financial arrangements by enabling equal access, an independent assessment of care needs, greater consumer choice, central and structured registration schemes for providers, and a well-trained care workforce (McCallum and Rees, 2017; Fine and Davidson, 2018). Two levels of support are available and delivered through government-approved providers: 1. Commonwealth Home Support Programme (CHSP): 75 per cent government subsidy for those aged 65 years and over requiring entry-level support services, including meals delivered, cleaning services, home maintenance/modifications, basic aids/equipment (for example, shower chair, bed hoist, walking aids) and community transport; and 2. Home Care Packages (HCPs) offering a personal budget for older adults with more complex and/or intensive care needs where a coordinated approach to the delivery of care services and assistance with everyday tasks is required (Department of Health, 2021a).

Aged Care Assessment Teams assess a person's needs and approve care provision through HCPs, residential care, transitional care, respite care and/or CHSP as required (Department of Health, 2021a). In 2018–19, aged care services in Australia were delivered to approximately 1.3 million people through CHSP (~840,000), residential aged care (~243,000) and HCPs (~133,000) (Royal Commission into Aged Care Quality and Safety, 2021a: 63). A National Priority System is in place to ensure allocation of HCPs is seen to be an equitable one, that is, allocated based on assessed need and circumstances irrespective of where an individual lives. However, it has been highlighted that the range of services available under the CHSP varies according to state and territory (Royal Commission into Aged Care Quality and Safety, 2021a).

Home Care Packages

Under the reforms, needs-based and means-tested[1] (income + assets) HCPs replaced high-intensity Community Care Packages; these were fully implemented for existing and new clients by 2015. Packages provide a personal budget to purchase a range of services to support health, well-being and independence, a safe and secure home environment, and social and community engagement. Services include allied health and therapy services, transport and personal assistance, telehealth, and assistive technology, aids and equipment. There are four HCP support levels allocated based on need: Level 1 (basic) ~AU$9,000 per annum/AU$25 per day to Level 4 (high care) ~AU$52,000 per annum/AU$144 per day (Department of Health, 2021a). The main access point for information and to initiate the process of assessment and allocation of packages is through the government's My Aged Care web-based portal. The most recent HCP Program Data Report released in June 2021 (Department of Health, 2021b) shows waiting times by HCP level (Table 3.1).

Home Care Package data

Available data from the Australian Government (Department of Health, 2021b) for the quarter ending 31 March 2021 indicate that the system of allocation, access and costs associated with

HCPs is under pressure in processing approvals, releasing additional packages and managing the National Priority System. The data reveal long waiting lists and a widening gap between assessment, approval and accessing a package. For example, in that quarter, 55,483 older adults seeking a package were not offered one; 31,679 were offered a lower level package (for example, Level 2) than their approved level (for example, Level 4); and of the 87,162 waiting for HCPs at their approved level, 98.8 per cent were provided the opportunity to connect to some form of subsidised home care support (for example, CHSP).

Table 3.1: Waiting times for HCPs, third quarter 2020–2021

Package level	Time to approved package
Level 1	3–6 months
Level 2	9–12 months
Level 3	9–12 months
Level 4	9–12 months

Source: Department of Health (2021b)

In 2019–2020, AU$21.5 billion was spent on aged care services: ~63 per cent on residential aged care; ~31 per cent on home care and support services; and ~5 per cent on community care services (for example, community nursing) (AIHW, 2021). In 2018–2019, personal contributions from recipients (see 'Home care packages' above) to overall revenue included HCP 4 per cent, CHSP 9 per cent and residential care 27 per cent (AIHW, 2021).

Evaluation of the reforms to date

The first legislated review of the reforms (Department of Health, 2017) reveals an uneven implementation with major concerns around the cost of administrative fees, lack of equity in access, extensive waiting lists, complexity of available information, and misalignment of client expectations, needs and available services (Department of Health, 2017). Clients' concerns included the lack of quality in available care services, reliance on/access issues related to the My Aged Care online portal, lack of information around choice in provider and services, staffing problems (for example, unavailable, lack of continuity) and cost of providers' administrative fees (McCallum and Rees, 2017; Batchelor et al 2020).

Small-scale studies from a provider perspective found that limited and rigid funding is insufficient to meet clients' goals, and heavy caseloads, administrative processes and waiting lists are overwhelming. Further concerns include lack of funding for infrastructure and limited resources for staff training (Davis et al, 2016; McCallum and Rees, 2017). These were particularly apparent in smaller, not-for-profit provider organisations, or those who served a specific client base such as rural communities, Indigenous Australians, or culturally and linguistically diverse communities.

The Final Report of Australia's Royal Commission into Aged Care Quality and Safety (2021) confirmed many of the concerns outlined above and concluded that Australia's aged care system remains difficult to access and navigate for older people and their families/carers; there are issues around equitable access, including long waiting lists and many service shortfalls; and there are ongoing problems in recruiting and retaining the care workforce. Of particular interest here, the report notes '*the care sector lags behind other sectors in the use and application of technology*' (Royal Commission into Aged Care Quality and Safety, 2021a: 77).

Technology and care policy and practice in Australia

Parallel to the CDC reforms in Australia is the increasing suggestion of technology to support ageing in place from governments (Barnett et al, 2017) and the health, medical and gerontechnology communities (National Aged Care Alliance, 2018; Australian Healthcare Associates, 2020). This is not unexpected given the predicted cost benefit and exponential rate in which new technologies are emerging and being integrated into society (Layton and Irlam, 2018; Australian Healthcare Associates, 2020). HCPs allow for the purchase of technologies, assistive devices and telehealth to assist ageing in place, suggesting the importance of such technologies for ageing well at home.

Defining technologies

Many technologies are available to support older adults. Some are considered everyday or mainstream technologies that are readily available and commonly used in society. Examples include mobile phones and microwave ovens. Others are considered assistive technologies, which are defined as any device or system aimed at maintaining or improving an individual's function and participation (Australian Association of Gerontology Assistive Technology Special Interest Group, 2020). Assistive technologies can be categorised in different ways. For example, in Australia, assistive technologies may encompass:

- manual technologies/aids/equipment (for example, walking frames, grips, rails, adaptors, hearing/visual aids);
- electronic aids/equipment (for example, hoists, mobile apps, home monitoring devices, GPS location/tracking devices);
- robotics (for example, assistive robots for lifting/medicine delivery, exoskeletons, social robots to create conversation, robots as social companions, service robots for health monitoring/surveillance/security, fall/gait detection);
- digital health technologies (for example, smart home technologies, telehealth, monitoring systems, communication aids/virtual assistants) (Australian Association of Gerontology Assistive Technology Special Interest Group, 2020).

Assistive technologies have also been categorised according to their level of complexity and the support required:

- low-risk technologies are simple, low-cost daily living aids/ support generally available to purchase (for example, pill organiser, landline telephone);
- under-advice technologies are generally available but usually require professional advice for safe/correct installation/use (for example, home modifications [ramps, rails], personal alarms, wheeled walker, shower chair);
- prescribed technologies are more complex/expensive technologies configured to meet individual support needs and typically involve allied health professional advice (for example, electric wheelchair, lifter chair, adjustable beds) (Australian Healthcare Associates, 2020).

A range of assistive technologies can be purchased using HCPs providing they support the care needs and personal goals of the older adult and facilitate health, well-being, safety and independence. Assistive technologies typically available within HCPs include basic continence aids (for example, commode chairs), mobility equipment (for example, wheeled walkers, wheelchairs, hoists, bed rails), communication aids (for example, hearing aids, telephone systems), personal care equipment (for example, shower chairs, toilet aids) and technologies to support telehealth services (Australian Government Department of Health, 2021). There are, however, differences in provision available in practice according to the state and territory, with the Royal Commission into Aged Care Quality and Safety (2021b) highlighting that South Australia has almost as many people accessing assistive technology as the rest of the other States and Territories combined. The report argues the complexity of various State and Territory assistive technology and home modification provision has 'resulted in a complex patchwork of supports' (the Royal Commission into Aged Care Quality and Safety, 2021b: 65).

As noted earlier, the Royal Commission into Aged Care Quality and Safety (2021a) also reported on the limited use of technology in aged care, and specifically mentioned the need for Australia's home care services to incorporate and implement a more clearly defined assistive technology and home modifications programme to support independence and safety of older people in the home (p 100). Indeed, the second volume of the report noted 'it is concerning that investment in home modification and assistive technology has declined so significantly under the Home Care Packages Program' (Royal Commission into Aged Care Quality and Safety, 2021b: 65), highlighting that when HCPs include technologies, the most popularly purchased items were washing machines (18 per cent of purchases) and televisions (17 per cent), and there was a significant decline in both the number and range of equipment previously accessed prior to the introduction of the HCP (Royal Commission into Aged Care Quality and Safety, 2021b).

There is also acknowledgement that the availability of devices is only part of the puzzle; it is also recommended that the provision of assistive technologies should be supported by services that help older adults select, obtain and use such technologies (Layton and Irlam, 2018). Selection of the most appropriate technology or combination of technologies, however, can be challenging (Haufe et al, 2019). While health professionals have a major role in this process, older adults and their families may develop their own simple technology solutions that better suit their individual circumstances (Bergschold et al, 2020).

Recent research evidence on technology and ageing in place in Australia

Empirical studies have considered the role and application of technology to support ageing in place in Australia. In their review, Layton and Irlam (2018) reported that many Australian older adults use a range of assistive technologies for self-care, mobility, communication, meal preparation and management of their health conditions. However, in practice in Australia, funding programmes are fragmented across different tiers of government and departments within those tiers.

There is growing recognition of the potential of technology to improve the lives of older adults in Australia (Layton and Irlam, 2018; National Aged Care Alliance, 2018; Australian Healthcare Associates, 2020) and internationally (Czaja, 2017). Potential benefits include:

- the promotion and support of healthy, active and independent living for older people;
- enablement of earlier health interventions and reablement strategies;
- enhanced social connections, increased confidence, participation and autonomy, and reduced anxiety;
- reduced carer stress and load;
- more cost-effective interventions, offsetting other health-related expenditure such as doctor visits or hospital admissions.

Assistive technology may improve the lives of older adults, particularly in areas such as physical well-being, safety, health monitoring, self-care and social connections (Layton and Irlam, 2018; National Aged Care Alliance, 2018; Australian Healthcare Associates, 2020). These areas are typically supported by allied health professionals such as occupational therapists and physiotherapists, social workers and community nurses, whose services are also accessible in Australia through HCPs (Department of Health, 2021a).

Although positive effects of technology have been reported in the literature (Khosravi and Ghapanchi, 2016), evidence of technology effectiveness from rigorously conducted evaluations such as controlled trials remains scarce (Ollevier et al, 2020), thus highlighting the need for more innovative approaches to generating this much needed evidence (Wang et al, 2021). How to best measure the efficacy of technology use to support ageing in place is also unclear (Pinto-Bruno et al, 2017). For older adults and service providers at least, technology for ageing in place can be considered successful if older adults' needs and wishes are prioritised, the technology is acceptable to the older adult and the technology provides benefits (Peek et al, 2016).

There are concerns that technology is not reaching its potential in older populations, despite its possible impact and general acceptability with those in mid to later life (Barnett et al, 2017). In their systematic review, Kapadia et al (2015) found many issues related to the implementation of technology in aged care, including misalignment between technology and workflow culture and service models, limited knowledge of available technology, insufficient funds, difficulties in understanding the role and possible benefits of potential technology, and the inconvenience of obtaining and using technology.

Although a reluctance by older adults to use technology has been reported as a barrier, such concerns can be overcome with appropriate training (Arthanet, 2021) or once technologies are trialled and the intended benefits realised (Ghorayeb et al, 2021). While the use of smart technologies has been commonly suggested as a way of supporting ageing in place, affordability, the right to privacy and dignity, and the ability to better customise such technologies remain a concern (Tural et al, 2021).

Australia's introduction of a CDC/personal budget model of funding of aged care incorporated the use of technology to support ageing in place and, from a health and social care perspective, a focus on delivering client-centred services. Taken individually, both these approaches have known shortcomings in their implementation; however, what is less clear is how the two systems are expected to be integrated in practice. Some frameworks have been developed in Australia for costing digital technologies that support ageing in place (Rahman et al, 2019).

However, if technology has some benefits for supporting ageing in place, and HCPs allow for purchasing devices to meet needs, how does this translate into practice from the perspective of the provider, the health and care professionals who work with the clients, and the clients and carers themselves?

The Older Adults' Use of Technology to Successfully Age in Place Project

To investigate these issues, we developed the Older Adults' Use of Technology to Successfully Age in Place Project. Our aims were to: 1. understand the national legislative/policy framework and provisions under a CDC funding model to support ageing in place; 2. explore the perceived impact of technology use on independence, participation, quality of life, social life and care needs of people ageing in place; and 3. explore how allied health professionals use technology as an intervention with older adults to improve ageing in place and how ageing in place outcomes are measured.

Study 1. Using technology to age in place: perspectives of older adults (Lovarini et al, 2019a)

In this first study, we interviewed 15 older adults receiving services from an aged care service provider and using technology related to health, housing, daily living, communication, leisure, mobility or transport. Most participants were aged over 75 years and more than half were female. Most lived in a house with about half the participants living on their own. Two thirds of participants received Level 3 or Level 4 HCPs. Participants used a range of mostly non-digital technologies (for example, personal alarms, electric lifter chairs, televisions, wheeled walkers, landline phone, shower aids). Fewer than half of the participants used smartphones, computers/laptops or streaming services.

The technology used by participants provided a range of benefits. Technology provided physical assistance; enhanced independence to reduce negative outcomes such as going into residential aged care; contributed to financial independence; provided psychological support and cognitive benefits; and helped participants feel good about themselves. Technology also supported meaningful activities such as involvement in charity work. Irrespective of the technology used, all participants needed support in technology selection, use and management. Support came mostly from family, friends and the aged care service provider, with few participants reporting involvement of allied health professionals.

From our investigation, we concluded that the technologies used by participants were mostly traditional, low risk, low tech and used for communicating with others, for entertainment and to support independence in activities of daily living. The combination of technologies differed across participants and was highly individualised. Technology was valued when it supported the goals and interests of the participants. Digital technology use was limited, and while a range of supports were needed for successful technology use, the role of allied health professionals in providing this support was not clear.

Study 2. Older adults and digital technologies (Lovarini et al, 2019b)

Informed by the findings from Study 1, we then identified and described key policy documents, reports and research to determine older adults' use of digital technologies and examined key studies focusing on technology for health and ageing in place. Drawing on data current at the time (Australian Communications and Media Authority, 2016), we found that 71 per cent of Australian adults aged over 65 were already using the Internet, with 85 per cent of older Internet users going online once a day for an average time of 7 hours per week. Desktop computer use was most common, but the use of tablets and mobile devices was increasing. The most common online activities were emailing, Internet banking and paying bills, with 43 per cent of older Internet users on social media.

Only 15 per cent used the Internet to access online government/health/medical services. In reviewing the international literature, we found that having a higher level of education, having a spouse/partner, a higher income and living in urban areas were all associated with Internet use by older adults. Personal factors were also important such as having a positive outlook, satisfaction with activities, being independent and persevering. Common reasons for non-use of digital technologies included having no interest or seeing no benefit, being too costly, and difficult to use, and a lack of confidence.

We identified a range of factors impacting on the use of technology for ageing in place. The widespread adoption of digital technologies by older people as a means of remaining independent at home was limited. Despite an increase in technology use by older people, not everyone had access to the Internet or broadband services in the home. Technology use was also less common among older cohorts, such as those aged over 80 years. Having enough knowledge and skills was critical not just for older adults but for families, other supporters and, in particular, health professionals who may not have considered digital technologies as a way of facilitating ageing in place outcomes for their older clients. Understanding the needs and preferences of older adults in relation to technology adoption and use was important. Support that is tailored to the individual needs, preferences and circumstances of the older adult was crucial whether that support came from family, peers, health professionals or from other service providers.

Our investigation highlighted the need for a greater understanding of the concerns of some older adults and their resistance to digital technology use; interventions likely to facilitate technology confidence, uptake and sustained use and services available for training; and ongoing support that suits the preferences and capacities of older adults. As with other aspects of care arrangements, having this understanding would ensure that older adults have greater choice, voice and control in the type, delivery and provision of technologies to support them to live independently, remain socially engaged and maintain their quality of life (Yeandle et al, 2012). These findings also suggested opportunities for allied health professionals to better support older adults. These include an acknowledgement and consideration of the digital literacy of their older clients; development of strategies to address client concerns and barriers to digital technology use; development and tailoring of interventions to enhance technology use; sourcing accessible and readily accessible technologies; and facilitating the sustained use of such technologies over time.

Study 3. Technology interventions used by allied health professionals to support ageing in place: a scoping review (Borilovic et al, 2019)

In this study, we conducted a scoping review to explore how allied health professionals use technology as an intervention with older adults to improve ageing in place and how ageing in place outcomes were measured. We searched 12 health databases for peer-reviewed intervention studies, published between 2008 and 2018, evaluating the effect of a technology that may be recommended by an allied health professional on ageing in place-related outcomes. Publications retrieved from the searches were independently screened and assessed for inclusion in the review. We conducted a narrative synthesis to summarise and compare study findings.

Forty-seven studies were included. The most commonly reported technologies were exergames (fitness games; n= 12, 26 per cent), telehealth/assistance (n=8, 17 per cent) and individual monitoring systems (n=5, 11 per cent). Almost all of the studies (n=46, 98 per cent) focused on one type of technological device or system. Intervention length varied from two weeks to 12 months, with 16 (34 per cent) studies lasting three months or longer and four (6 per cent) studies conducting interventions for 12 months.

Technology was commonly used as a therapeutic device to improve physical or emotional conditions (such as poor balance or loneliness), an assistive device to provide support with common problematic tasks (such as taking medicine), or a monitoring device on the older person's health and safety. Person-centred approaches to technology use were limited to four (9 per cent) studies only. In these studies, participants chose their own goals for technology use in collaboration with the researcher and had a say in when and how they were taught to use the technology. In each of these four studies, the intervention involved one-on-one coaching between the researcher and the participant (and sometimes their carer) and was individualised for the participant to achieve their goal. Fifteen studies (32 per cent) included training where the participant could practice using the technology prior to the intervention. Almost half of the studies (n=23, 49 per cent) did not specify how the technology was implemented, by whom or if there were any instructions involved. While 20 different ageing in place-related outcomes were reported in the included studies, there were inconsistencies in the outcome measures used and how ageing in place outcomes were defined. The most common outcomes were well-being and quality of life (n=26, 43 per cent), fall-related outcomes (n=23, 19 per cent), and activity- and task-related outcomes (n=20, 42 per cent).

The impact of the COVID-19 pandemic and the importance of co-design

The findings from our three studies and the broader literature highlight the importance of person-centred approaches for the development, implementation and evaluation of technologies for ageing in place (Ollevier et al, 2020). Since our project, a key influence on the use of technology, especially digital technologies, by older adults has been the COVID-19 pandemic. Challenges faced by older adults over the pandemic period have included decreased social interactions, reduced quality of life, increased depression, difficulties accessing services, reduced physical activity and unmet service need for assistance with activities of daily living (Lebrasseur et al,

2021). The pandemic has also highlighted the importance of digital literacy for older adults with the increasing reliance on digital technologies and services. Pleasingly, there has been an increase in the use of digital technologies by older adults over the pandemic period internationally (Daly et al, 2021) and in Australia (Strutt et al, 2021). Despite this positive outcome, the impact of the pandemic on supportive care environments and digital technologies has been identified as a key research priority (Rylett et al, 2020), while disruptions to the provision of assistive technology during the pandemic has also led to calls for more user-centred systems that are flexible, resilient and sustainable (Smith et al, 2020).

To achieve this goal, partnerships between older adults, allied health professionals, service providers and governments are needed. Co-design of technologies, interventions to enhance technology use and evaluation of impact may provide a way forward. Definitions vary but co-design generally refers to the collaborative involvement of users, designers, providers and procurers in the development of services (Sumner et al, 2020). In their comprehensive review of studies investigating co-design of technologies for ageing in place, Sumner and colleagues found that the co-design process varied across studies and few studies reported on the health and well-being impact of using a co-design approach. Others have also reported that while older adults are keen to be involved in the co-design process (Wang et al, 2019), it currently remains unclear whether co-design approaches lead to enhanced acceptance, adoption and use of technology by older adults (Fischer et al, 2020). Living Labs have been proposed as a way of enhancing the co-design process (Knight-Davidson et al, 2020), with Living Labs operating in Europe[2] and Australia.[3]

Conclusion

There is a growing focus in Australia on the importance of technology for ageing in place, and policies, funding packages and services have been developed to support this goal. The provision of HCPs to support older adults to remain living in their own homes provides a personal budget that can be applied in purchasing a range of services, including allied health and therapy services, telehealth and assistive technology, aids and equipment. Despite these advances and the availability of technologies, access to and use of technology for ageing in place remains fragmented and inequitable, and, where it is available, presents as a challenge for many older Australians and their families/carers. Our programme of research has highlighted the importance of tailored, individualised, sustained support for older adults along with key strategies that allied health professionals can use to facilitate such support. We recommend co-design approaches as a way of progressing research on this topic to ensure that technology for ageing in place is truly person-centred.

Acknowledgements

We acknowledge the contribution of Associate Professor Ann-Helen Patomella (Karolinska Institutet), Dr Sanetta du Toit (The University of Sydney), Professor Sue Yeandle (University of Sheffield) and Jacinta Borilovic (The University of Sydney) to The Older Adults' Use of Technology to Successfully Age in Place Project and, in particular, Jacinta's input into the scoping review.

We would also like to acknowledge The University of Sydney for making available the Ageing in Place Seeding Grant (2017–2019), and the Australian Research Council Centre of Excellence in Population Ageing Research (CE170100005) for their ongoing support of our contribution to the ESRC research programme Sustainable Care: connecting people and systems, 2017–21 (ES/P009255/1).

Notes

1 Full pensioners (for example, age, veterans) and those with an annual income below AU$28,472.60 are exempt from an income assessment.

In the income range AU$28,472.60–54,990, a daily fee of AU$15.81 up to AU$31.63 applies and is deducted from the government subsidy for HCPs; annual and lifetime caps apply on income-tested fees. Owning your home is not included in the assets test. Further details can be accessed at https://www.myagedcare.gov.au/home-care-package-costs-and-fees#what- do-i-pay

2 https://enoll.org/

3 https://www.gcma.net.au/modern-ageing-living-laboratory-network-na

References

Arthanet, S. (2021) 'Promoting information communication technology adoption and acceptance for aging-in-place: a randomized controlled trial', *Journal of Applied Gerontology,* 40(5): 471–480.

Australian Association of Gerontology Assistive Technology Special Interest Group. (2020) 'Assistive Technology SIG (TECHSIG)'. Available at: https://www.aag.asn.au/education/special-interest-groups/assistive-technology-sig-techsig [accessed 21.04.22].

Australian Communications and Media Authority. (2016) 'Digital lives of older Australians'. Canberra, Commonwealth of Australia.

Australian Government Department of Health. (2021) 'Home care packages program. Operational manual for home care package consumers. Version 1.2'. Available at: https://www.myagedcare.gov.au/sites/default/files/2021-09/operational-manual-for-home-care-package-consumers.pdf [accessed 25.11.22].

Australian Healthcare Associates. (2020) 'Review of Assistive Technology Programs in Australia', final report for the Australian Government Department of Health. Available at: https://www.health.gov.au/sites/default/files/documents/2021/02/review-of-assistive-technology-programs-in-australia-final-report_0.pdf [accessed 25.11.22].

Australian Institute of Health and Welfare [AIHW]. (2021) 'GEN Fact Sheet 2019–20: Spending on aged care', Canberra: AIHW.

Barnett, K., Reynolds, K., Gordon, S., Hobbs, D. and Maeder, A. (2017) 'Developing a technology roadmap for the Australian aged care sector: literature review'. Available at: https://aciitc.com.au/wp-content/uploads/2017/06/ACIITC_TechnologyRoadmapLiteratureReview_2017.pdf [accessed 25.11.22].

Batchelor, F., Savvas, S., Peck, A., Dang, C., Wade, C., Goh, A.M.Y., et al (2020) 'Inside the system: home and respite care clients' perspectives', Parkville, Victoria, Australia: National Ageing Research Institute. Available at: https://agedcare.royalcommission.gov.au/sites/default/files/2020-10/research-paper-14.pdf [accessed 23.02.23].

Bergschold, J.M., Neven, L. and Peine, A. (2020) 'DIY gerontechnology: circumventing mismatched technologies and bureaucratic procedure by creating care technologies of one's own', *Sociology of Health and Illness*, 42(2): 232–246.

Borilovic, J., Lovarini, M., Clemson, L. and O'Loughlin, K. (2019) 'What are they doing and what are they measuring? A scoping review on the technological interventions and ageing in place outcomes allied health professionals use'. Paper presented at Association for the Advancement of Assistive Technology in Europe Conference, 15th International Conference: Global Challenges in Assistive Technology: Research, Policy and Practice, Bologna, Italy. Available at: https://aaate2019.eu/wp-content/uploads/sites/24/2019/08/AAATE2019_Proceedings.pdf [accessed 25.11.22].

Czaja, S. (2017) 'The potential role of technology in supporting older adults', *Public Policy and Aging Report*, 27(2): 44–48.

Daly, J.R., Depp, C., Graham, S.A., Jeste, D.V., Kim, H., Lee, E., et al (2021) 'Health impacts of the Stay-at-Home Order on community-dwelling older adults and how technologies may help: focus group study', *JMIR Aging*, 4(1): e25779.

Davis, J., Morgans, A., Birks, M. and Browning, C. (2016) 'The rhetoric and reality of nursing in aged care: views from the inside', *Contemporary Nurse*, 52(2–3): 191–203.

Department of Health. (2017) 'Legislated review of aged care 2017'. Available at: https://www.health.gov.au/sites/default/files/legislated-review-of-aged-care-2017-report.pdf [accessed 25.11.22].

Department of Health. (2021a) 'Home Care Packages'. Available at: https://www.myagedcare.gov.au/help-at-home/home-care-packages [accessed 25.11.22].

Department of Health. (2021b) 'Home care packages program data report, 3rd quarter 2020-21'. Available at: https://www.gen-agedcaredata.gov.au/www_aihwgen/media/Home_care_report/Home-Care-Data-Report-3rd-Qtr-2020-21.pdf [accessed 24.01.23].

Fine, M. and Davidson, B. (2018) 'The marketization of care: global challenges and national responses in Australia', *Current Sociology Monograph*, 66(4): 503–516.

Fischer, B., Peine, A. and Östlund, B. (2020) 'The importance of user involvement: a systematic review of involving older users in technology design', *The Gerontologist*, 60(7): e513–e523.

Ghorayeb, A., Comber, R. and Gooberman-Hill, R. (2021) 'Older adults' perspectives of smart home technology: are we developing the technology that older people want?' *International Journal of Human–Computer Studies*, 147: 102571.

Haufe, M., Theodorus, S., Peek, M. and Luijkx, K. (2019) 'Matching gerontechnologies to independent-living seniors' individual needs: development of the GTM tool', *BMC Health Services Research*, 19(26).

Kapadia V., Ariani A., Li J. and Ray P.K. (2015) 'Emerging ICT implementation issues in aged care', *International Journal of Medical Informatics*, 84(11): 892–900.

Khosravi, P. and Ghapanchi, A.H. (2016) 'Investigating the effectiveness of technologies applied to assist seniors: a systematic literature review', *International Journal of Medical Informatics*, 85(1): 17–26.

Knight-Davidson, P., Lane, P. and McVicar, A. (2020) 'Methods for co-creating with older adults in living laboratories: a scoping review', *Health and Technology*, 10: 997–1009.

Layton, N. and Irlam, C. (2018) 'Assistive technology for older Australians: rapid evidence review and economic pathway analysis'. Available at: https://apo.org.au/node/262176 [accessed 18.01.23].

Lebrasseur, A., Fortin-Bédard, N., Lettre, J., Raymond, E., Bussieres, E-L., Lapierre, N., et al (2021) 'Impact of the COVID-19 pandemic on older adults: rapid review', *JMIR Aging*, 4(2): e26474.

Lovarini, M., O'Loughlin, K. and Clemson, L. (2019a) 'Older adults and digital technologies', in Attrill-Smith, A., Fullwood, C., Keep, M. and Kuss, D. (Eds) *The Oxford Handbook of Cyberpsychology*, Oxford: Oxford University Press.

Lovarini, M., O'Loughlin, K., Clemson, L. and Dickson, C. (2019b) 'Using technology to age in place: perspectives of older adults'. Presented at Occupational Therapy Australia 28th National Conference and Exhibition, Sydney, NSW, Australia. Available at: https://onlinelibrary.wiley.com/doi/epdf/10.1111/1440-1630.12585 [accessed 25.11.22].

McCallum, J. and Rees, K. (2017) 'Consumer directed care in Australia: early stage analysis and future directions', Brisbane: National Seniors. Available at: https://agedcare.royalcommission.gov.au/sites/default/files/2019-12/08172617par-consumer-directed-care-research-report-fnemail.pdf [accessed 21.02.23].

National Aged Care Alliance. (2018) 'Position paper: assistive technology for older Australians'. Available at: https://naca.asn.au/wp-content/uploads/2018/11/NACA_Assistive_Technology_for_Older_Australians_Position_Paper-1-June-2018.pdf [accessed 25.11.22].

Ollevier, A., Aguiar, G., Palomino, M. and Simpelaere, I.S. (2020) 'How can technology support ageing in place in healthy older adults? A systematic review', *Public Health Reviews,* 41: 26.

Peek, S.T.M., Wouters, E.J., Luijkx, K.G. and Vrijhoef H.J. (2016) 'What it takes to successfully implement technology for aging in place: focus groups with stakeholders', *Journal of Medical Internet Research*, 18(5): e98.

Pinto-Bruno, Á.C., García-Casal, J.A., Csipke, E., Jenaro-Río, C. and Franco-Martin, M. (2017) 'ICT-based applications to improve social health and social participation in older adults with dementia. A systematic literature review', *Aging and Mental Health*, 21(1): 58–65.

Productivity Commission (2011) 'Caring for older Australians: overview'. Report No. 53, Final Inquiry Report, Canberra. Available at: https://www.pc.gov.au/inquiries/completed/aged-care/report/aged-care-overview-booklet.pdf [accessed 25.11.22].

Rahman, A., Akbar, D., Rolfe, J. and Nguyen, J. (2019) 'Developing a population wide cost estimating framework and methods for technological intervention enabling ageing in place: an Australian case', *PLoS ONE*, 14(6): e0218448.

Royal Commission into Aged Care Quality and Safety (2021a) 'Final report - volume 1: summary and recommendations'. Commonwealth of Australia. Available at: https://agedcare.royalcommission.gov.au/publications/final-report-volume-1 [accessed 25.11.22].

Royal Commission into Aged Care Quality and Safety (2021b) 'Final report - volume 2: the current system'. Commonwealth of Australia. Available at: https://agedcare.royalcommission.gov.au/publications/final-report-volume-2 [accessed 25.11.22].

Rylett, R.J., Alary, F., Goldberg, J., Rogers, S. and Versteegh, P. (2020) 'COVID-19 and priorities for research in aging', *Canadian Journal on Aging*, 39(4): 500–505.

Smith, E., Toro Hernandez, M.L., Ebuenyi, I.D., Syurina, E., Barbareschi, G., Best, K., et al (2022) 'Assistive technology use and provision during COVID-19: results from a rapid global survey', *International Journal of Health Policy and Management*, 11(6): 747–756.

Strutt, P., Johnco, C., Chen, J., Muira, C., Mauricea, O., Dawes, P., et al (2022) 'Stress and coping in older Australians during COVID-19: health, service utilization, grandparenting, and technology use', *Clinical Gerontologist*, 45(1): 106–119.

Sumner, J., Chong, L.S., Bundele, A. and Lim, Y.W. (2021). 'Co-designing technology for aging in place: a systematic review', *The Gerontologist*, 61(7): e395–e409.

Tural, E., Lu, D. and Cole, D.A. (2021) 'Safely and actively aging in place: older adults' attitudes and intentions toward smart home technologies', *Aging and Technology*, 7: 1–15.

Wang, R., Kenyon, L., McGilton, K., Miller, W., Hovanec, N., Boger, J., et al (2021) 'The time is now: a FASTER approach to generate research evidence for technology-based interventions in the field of disability and rehabilitation', *Archives of Physical Medicine and Rehabilitation*, 102(9): 1848–1859.

Wang, S., Bolling, K., Mao, W., Reichstadt, J., Jeste, D., Kim, H-C., et al (2019) 'Technology to support aging in place: older adults' perspectives', *Healthcare*, 7(2): 60.

Yeandle, S., Kröger, T. and Cass, B. (2012) 'Voice and choice for users and carers? Developments in patterns of care for older people in Australia, England and Finland', *Journal of European Social Policy*, 22(4): 432–445.

FOUR

The role of assistive technologies in home care delivery in Germany: between vision and reality

Andreas Hoff and Bill Pottharst

Social care: policy, debates and evidence

Approach to and structure of social care

Long-term care (LTC) legislation in Germany rests on the traditional principles of a conservative–corporatist welfare state regime (Esping-Andersen, 1990) and a care regime reliant on unpaid care (though partly compensated for by the government) (Anttonen and Sipilä, 1996). There are increasing tensions between the assumption that families will take responsibility for LTC versus the country's societal reality of an ageing population and the changing of norms and values regarding family life and (female) labour market participation.

The Long-Term Care Insurance (LTCI), which was implemented in 1995 for home care and in 1996 for residential care (Bundestag, 1994), did not change the family's obligation to provide LTC – if anything, it reinforced it by adding a *legal* obligation to the moral obligation for families to provide care. The law explicitly states: 'LTCI is meant to support with their benefits primarily home care and the willingness of family members and neighbours to give care in order to allow those in need of care to stay in their homes for as long as possible' (Bundestag, 1994, authors' translation). LTC is thus geared towards care at home, which is in line with the expressed preference of the vast majority of Germans (80 per cent want to be cared for at home, see also Hayek et al, 2018; Kuhlmey et al, 2010).

Moreover, costs of home care for the state are significantly lower than those for residential care (BMG, 2021a). However, critics argue LTCI does not cover all care-related expenses regardless of care setting, leaving families to shoulder extra costs (for example, Hielscher et al, 2017). This focus on home care not only aligns with the traditional role of the family in German society; it also reflects the *subsidiarity* principle, which, when applied to LTC, means local authorities will step in if – but only if – the family is unable to cope. As such, LTCI was never meant to cover *all* expenses related to LTC (see section on 'Level of met/unmet need').

LTCI mirrors the health insurance (*Krankenversicherung* or 'sickness insurance') in that everybody living in Germany is obliged to take out both types of insurance, either in the statutory (as 89 per cent of the population do) or private system (11 per cent of people) (BMG, 2021a). LTCI is administered by 'LTC funds' (*Pflegekassen*) established under the existing umbrella of the 'health insurance funds' (*Krankenkassen*). LTCI benefit amounts are calculated according to care need and care arrangement (home care vs residential care), corresponding to an LTC grade. Access to LTC benefits expanded significantly following a major LTCI reform in 2017, with two main changes: 1. the equalisation of care need caused by dementia to a physical disability; and 2. the replacement of the previous three LTC degrees (*Pflegestufen*) with five distinct LTC grades (*Pflegegrade*). Instead of the previous approach of calculating the amount of time in minutes needed for caregiving, the 'need of care' (*Pflegebedürftigkeit*) is now determined by the degree of an individual's autonomy, independence, impairments or incapacitation in six fields (modules), which are weighted as follows: mobility (10 per cent); cognitive and communicative abilities, behaviour patterns and psychological problems (15 per cent); level of self-sufficiency (40 per cent); health restrictions, demands and stress due to therapies (20 per cent); and structure of everyday life and social contacts (15 per cent). The grade of care is determined by the Medical Services of the Statutory Health Insurance Funds (*Medizinischer Dienst der Gesetzlichen Krankenkassen*) or by its private counterpart (EC, 2021; Jacobs et al, 2021). Above grade 1, cash payments to informal caregivers are always considerably lower than payments for professional carers (Table 4.1). It is possible to combine them.

Cash payments for respite care (*Verhinderungspflege*) (up to six weeks per year) or short-term care (*Kurzzeitpflege*) (up to eight weeks per year) are not included in Table 4.1. Furthermore, residents in sheltered accommodation are entitled to a monthly supplement of €214. Moreover, working carers are entitled to ten working days of care support payment (*Pflegeunterstützungsgeld*) to organise care (BMG, 2022).

Table 4.1: LTCI benefit payments per month by grade and type of care (in euros)

LTCI grade	LTCI benefit for informal care per month	LTCI for formal home care per month	LTCI for residential care per month
Grade 1	€125	€125	€125
Grade 2	€316	€724	€770
Grade 3	€545	€1,363	€1,262
Grade 4	€728	€1,693	€1,775
Grade 5	€901	€2,095	€2,005

Source: BMG, 2022, using the German country profile in the European Commission's long-term care report 2021 (EC, 2021) as a template for translating the German LTCI terminology into English

Social care: key statistics

Population ageing

Germany is an advanced ageing society, with 21.5 per cent (EC, 2021) of its total population of 83 million aged 65 years and over, 11.4 per cent aged 75 years or older (EC, 2021) and 2.8 per cent aged 85 years and over (Eurostat, 2020). The risk of needing LTC rises with age from 1.6 per cent for those under 60 years to 8 per cent for people aged 60 to 80 years, reaching 39.9 per cent for those older than 80 years (BMG, 2021a).

Numbers of older adults receiving social care

Nearly 4.6 million people receive LTCI benefits at present, with more than 80 per cent (3.7 million) receiving home care and the remainder (900,000) in residential care (BMG, 2021a). These figures underestimate real demand for care due to the eligibility requirements for LTCI benefits; it is estimated as many as 5.8 million people require LTC in Germany (EC, 2021).

In 2020, of those who received LTCI for home care, nearly half (45.2 per cent) received LTC grade 2 benefits (the lowest grade that qualifies for professional care), a quarter (26.9 per cent) received LTC grade 3 (the middle category), 15.4 per cent qualified for the lowest degree of social care (LTC grade 1), and 9.3 per cent received benefits LTC grade 4 and 3.2 per cent LTC grade 5 (that is, the highest categories). In contrast, higher LTC grades dominate among residential care recipients. The equivalent figures for private LTCI are similar (BMG, 2021a).

Expenditure for long-term care

Total expenditure on statutory LTCI is equivalent to 1.6 per cent of Germany's gross domestic product (EC, 2021) and amounted to €45.6 billion in 2020 – €29.1 billion for home care and €16.5 billion for residential care (BMG, 2021a).

Expenditure more than doubled within the past decade, caused by rising numbers of people requiring LTC, as well as a substantial increase of people eligible to receive LTCI benefits following the 2017 reform. Currently, 40.8 per cent of total LTC public expenditure is spent on cash benefits, 35.7 per cent on residential care and 23.5 per cent on home care (EC, 2021).

Level of met/unmet need

At the societal level, there was a deficit of several 100 million euros during the majority of the early/mid-2000s that shifted to a slight surplus until the mid-2010s following the 2008 LTCI reform. In 2017 and 2018, substantial deficits of €2.4 billion and €3.55 billion, respectively, occurred, possibly a temporary effect of expanding the number of people eligible for LTCI benefits following the 2017 reform. The figures for 2019 and 2020 were more favourable (BMG, 2021a), though the full effect of the COVID-19 pandemic was not included in these calculations.

At the individual level, there is substantial unmet need as LTCI was never intended to cover all expenses related to LTC. Families are required to cover costs that exceed the amount of LTCI from their own resources or private insurance cover (Althammer et al, 2021). A state-subsidised complementary insurance scheme (*private Pflegezusatzversicherung/Pflege-Bahr*) was introduced in 2012, but has low coverage (only 850,000 people) (Statista, 2020). Gaps between the LTCI and care need are common and increase as the person receiving care becomes more frail (Rothgang et al, 2020), with a means-tested LTCI benefit (*Hilfe zur Pflege*) available for those unable to afford additional coverage and only applicable to LTC grades 2 to 5.

Structure of social care workforce

It is almost impossible to talk about LTC in Germany without framing it as 'care crisis' (*Pflegekrise*) or 'care emergency' (*Pflegenotstand*), which refers to severe shortages in the care workforce. According to the Federal Employment Agency (*Bundesagentur für Arbeit*), there were 1.7 million care workers in 2020 – 1.1 million in healthcare and 615,000 in eldercare (Bundesagentur-für-Arbeit, 2021). This represents an increase of 2 per cent or 40,000 compared with the previous year (Bundesagentur-für-Arbeit, 2021), but is not nearly sufficient to close the gap between demand for care workers and supply.

Women are overrepresented: 80 per cent of healthcare workers and 83 per cent of eldercare workers are women. Furthermore, the share of part-time employment is unusually high in care professions: 43 per cent of healthcare workers and 55 per cent of eldercare workers are working part-time, which is substantially higher than in other professions. The number of migrant care workers increased over the same period by 31,000 to 84,000 (2020), almost equally divided between healthcare and eldercare (Bundesagentur-für-Arbeit, 2021).

Role of unpaid carers

Family or informal carers are commonly referred to as 'Germany's biggest care provider' (*Deutschlands größter Pflegedienst*), with nearly 70 per cent of those receiving statutory home care LTCI benefits (3.3 million) cared for by informal carers only (principally by family carers), with the remainder being looked after jointly by home care providers and family carers (Destatis, 2020). There are no official statistics on the numbers of people involved in informal or family caregiving. Research evidence cannot easily be compared due to the use of different definitions of care. Geyer (2016) estimated that as many as 6 per cent of the total population aged 16 to 64 provide care to a family member (4–5 million people) (Geyer, 2016; Unabhängiger-Beirat-Vereinbarkeit-Pflege-Beruf, 2019). The average weekly care commitment is estimated between 13.5 hours per week (Institut-DGB-Index-Gute-Arbeit, 2018) and 18 hours per week (Engstler and Tesch-Römer, 2017), but some primary caregivers provide care for up to 63 hours per week (Hielscher et al, 2017).

Social care and technology: policy and practice

In the Germany context, 'assistive technologies' in the past 20 years included mechanical devices, such as 'grabber' grip extensions, ramps and stairlifts, but also distress call buttons and memory aids. There has also been growing use of digital devices such as on networked control systems connecting sensors, computers and actors into complex cyber-physical systems, including smart homes, smartphones, tracking and navigation systems, and vitality and health apps. In addition, there is an increased proliferation of fourth generation technologies such as virtual reality, augmented reality, assisted driving aids, and robots to support care, emotions, household chores and socialisation. Recent technological advances in digitisation also include the use of 'Big Data', cloud computing, Internet of Things (IoT) devices, artificial intelligence (AI), machine learning and autonomous systems, as well as interactive and telepresence robots (Bundestag, 2020).

Whereas LTC is governed by legislation, technologies are only beginning to make their way into these frameworks. Unless digital solutions are officially authorised technologies by the LTC system, they are not eligible for compensation via LTCI. This is in sharp contrast to the high hopes policy makers place on digital technologies as part of the solution for 'the care crisis' in Germany as expressed in various statements, such as the following: '… the development and use of technology for life in old age is closely associated with the hope of improving the daily lives and provisioning of older people … It is also a driver of research and technological development' (Bundestag, 2020: 4; authors' translation).

Principles

There are several committees advising the German government on care-related issues, representing a variety of interest groups (family carers' and care professionals' lobbying organisations, trade unions, employers' associations, statutory/private health insurances/LTCI) and academics with relevant research expertise. Several in turn have highlighted the potential of digitisation for improving quality of life in old age but in contrast to the government, these committees have emphasised preconditions for a successful use of technology by older people and their carers (Unabhängiger-Beirat-Vereinbarkeit-Pflege-Beruf, 2019; Bundestag, 2020).

The best reference point for an independent position on key principles on technology and care is the 'Eighth Report on the Situation of the Older Generation in Germany' (*Achter Bundesaltenbericht*) (subsequently '8th Ageing Report') published in 2020 that focused on 'older people and digitisation' (Bundestag, 2020). Ageing Reports are of high significance and public visibility, presenting state-of-the-art reviews on specific age-related topics chosen by the German parliament and compiled by leading experts. The German parliament (*Deutscher Bundestag*) commissions a report focused on a different theme related to the situation of older people in each election period, and the 8th Ageing Report explored whether digitisation could enhance older people's circumstances and highlighted opportunities related to autonomy and independent living. The key principles included in the 8th Ageing Report are outlined in Box 4.1.

BOX 4.1: KEY PRINCIPLES OF THE 8TH AGEING REPORT

- Digitisation has to be considered in relation to scientific knowledge in gerontology to recognise its impact on cognitive, emotional, social and physical ageing.
- Digitisation has to be discussed in the context of person–environment interactions against the background of social inequality and the plurality of life worlds and lifestyles in old age.
- By considering social inequality, the existence and causes of a 'digital divide' in society are recognised.
- Digital sovereignty of older people is crucial for success.
- There are tensions between the needs of older people on the one hand and the dynamics of digitisation on the other.
- Digitisation has to be negotiated at individual, organisational and societal levels.

- Both opportunities and risks of digitisation, as well as ethical implications, have to be considered.
- An interdisciplinary approach to digitisation is important.

The report discusses opportunities for improving older people's quality of life by using digital technologies in areas such as stimulation and activation, maintaining social networks and improving social participation, compensatory enhancement in cases of sensory, motor or cognitive impairments. Another promising theme is the introduction of digital patient records replacing the previous paper-based files, which is presented as a milestone in giving people more control over documentation of their patient history and medication. Telemedicine and telehealth are seen as means for overcoming time and spatial constraints in rural areas in particular, and videoconferencing or telemonitoring applications for monitoring chronic conditions, such as cardiac function. Furthermore, the report cites the 'First Report of the Independent Committee for the Reconciliation of Caregiving and Employment' (*Unabhängiger Beirat für die Vereinbarung von Pflege und Beruf*), stressing the potential of technology for improving the reconciliation of caregiving and employment (Unabhängiger-Beirat-Vereinbarkeit-Pflege-Beruf, 2019).

At the heart of the 8th Ageing Report is human–technology interaction, with a specific focus on older people. Acceptance of digital technologies by its intended users and their competency in using technology is crucial for success. Data protection and privacy are covered extensively since concern about infringement of the latter has previously been a major obstacle to a greater technology uptake. More specifically, the report discusses the use and protection of personal data, the risks of data sharing in a networked society and the need for global regulation of globally operating digital companies. According to the report, the extraordinary dynamic development of new digital technologies prevents a (thorough) risk analysis prior to marketisation of digital products and services. The authors of the report suggest strengthening responsibility and 'digital sovereignty' of individual users/consumers as the best way forward to meet this challenge (Bundestag, 2020).

Policy

The 8th Ageing Report is a highly influential report advising German policy makers. The most important player in shaping LTC policy is the Federal Ministry of Health (*Bundesministerium für Gesundheit*), which is in charge of LTCI. It is also responsible for the 2008 and 2015 Caregiver Leave Act (*Pflegezeitgesetz*), whereas another central government department – the Federal Ministry for Families, Senior Citizens, Women and Youth (*Bundesministerium für Familie, Senioren, Frauen und Jugend*) – is in charge of the 2012 and 2015 Family Caregiver Leave Act (*Familienpflegezeitgesetz*) (BMFSFJ, 2021). However, it is unclear who is in charge of digitisation and ageing. Here, two other central government departments come into play, neither of them responsible for either LTC/health care or older people: the Federal Ministry for Economic Affairs and Energy (*Bundesministerium für Wirtschaft und Energie*) and the Federal Ministry of Education and Research (*Bundesministerium für Bildung und Forschung* [BMBF]).

The key player in strategic research planning is the central government department responsible for research development, making available several billion euros per year for research. Its recommendations on future research are the closest Germany gets to a strategy on digital development. The following statement on the Ministry's homepage states its mission and self-perception as focused on 'academic excellence' with a strategy of 'comprehensive interdepartmental innovation strategy' and the identification and establishment of 'new research themes and ... new instruments of innovation facilitation' (BMBF, 2021, authors' translation). The government's strategy on research and development on technology for older people/LTC has its origins in three different central government strategies: 1. its strategy on tackling the challenges resulting from 'demographic change'; 2. its 'high-tech strategy'; and 3. its 'digitisation strategy' that specifies the 'high-tech strategy' in regard to digitisation.

The 'demographic change' strategy

In 1992, the German parliament established a committee of enquiry (*Enquete Kommission*) to inform the *Bundestag* on imminent population ageing and its consequences for German society. In 2009, its first 'demography strategy' was published, followed by the publication of the government's first 'Demography Report' in 2011. A series of high-profile events related to the demography strategy has taken place almost on an annual basis ever since (BiB, 2021). The strategy aims to address four central objectives: 1. to strengthen economic growth; 2. to facilitate social cohesion; 3. to promote equal living conditions in all regions of the country; and 4. to maintain solid public finances.

The facilitation of the demographic change strategy was accompanied by the '2013 Science Year on Demographic Opportunities' (*Wissenschaftsjahr zur demographischen Chance*), which started a central government campaign identifying opportunities in demographic change, rather than population ageing being a burden on German society and the German economy (BMBF, 2013). Most relevant in the context of this chapter was a positive campaign under the headings 'Experiences and Perspectives' and 'Lifelong Learning' introducing thematic streams such as 'health and long-term care', 'a better life with technology' and 'being out and about thanks to technology'. The focus of the latter was on technology in housing, social robotics in dementia care and the 2013 BMBF programme entitled 'Senior Technology Ambassadors' of older people engaging in peer-to-peer digital technology training, which, though considered a hugely successful programme, was not extended after the initial funding period expired. We consider it notable that the '2013

Science Year on Demographic Opportunities' was followed by the '2014 Science Year on Digital Society'.

The German 'High-Tech Strategy 2025'

Germany's 'High-Tech Strategy 2025' was published in 2018 (BMBF, 2018a, 2018b). In its introductory statement, the German government outlines its vision: 'Only with excellent research and the effective transfer ... into practical application will we be able to find creative answers to the grand challenges and strengthen our economy in times of ever-faster change and ever-tougher global competition' (BMBF, 2018b: 4). Germany's high-tech strategy focuses on three major objectives, the first of which is 'tackling grand challenges', with digitisation presented as a key solution related to a) health and care; b) sustainability, climate protection and energy; c) mobility; d) urban and rural areas; e) safety and security; and f) economy and work. It is noteworthy that 'health and care' is mentioned first in the list of topics. Most relevant for future development of technology in LTC is the drive for digitalisation in preventive and personalised care and nursing care devices, '... with the aim of relieving the workload of nursing staff and relatives, giving them more time for human attention and improving the quality of life of those in need of care' (BMBF, 2018b: 18). A closer look reveals that priority is given to healthcare and the medical sphere (telemedicine, 'intelligent medicine', cancer treatment, and so on). However, residential care is part of a new 'Future of Care Cluster' introduced in 2018 in which '... research and industry are working together with users on new products, processes and methods to improve everyday nursing care in Germany for all those involved. Social and technical innovations are to be closely interlinked in this process' (BMBF, 2018b: 19).

The second objective focuses on strengthening Germany's future competencies through the systematic development of 'key enabling technologies' aiming at 'disruptive innovation potential', with AI as a dominant theme. Two new funding streams highly relevant for the development of technologies are introduced here, albeit under the headings of 'Societal participation' and 'Using the potential of the social sciences': 1. the ethical, legal and social implications network for human–machine interaction; and 2. the establishment of a Data Ethics Commission addressing the right to informational self-determination. The final objective refers to establishing an open innovation and venture culture, focused on 'creativity, agility and openness to new ideas', and identifies start-ups and small and medium-sized enterprises as the most important actors in achieving this; it is thus relevant since the majority of technology developers in Germany are small and medium-sized companies.

In 2021, the government reviewed the 'High-Tech Strategy' (BMBF, 2021). In the wake of the COVID-19 pandemic, health protection has moved centre stage. Research on health in general and more specifically research on prevention, diagnosis and therapy of COVID-19 are hailed for their crucial role during the pandemic. But the COVID-19 pandemic has also resulted in a much greater focus in German society on widespread deficits in social care. This is also reflected in the review of the 'High-Tech Strategy' that now explicitly mentions (assistive) technology as key element of the future strategy on LTC: 'Future social care will be supported by assistive technologies and digital solutions, which will be oriented on the needs of care recipients, professional carers and care-giving family members' (BMBF, 2021: 19, authors' translation). Two new research funding programmes were established: 1. 'Innovations in LTC 2030', focusing on both new technologies in LTC and quality of life of formal/informal carers; and 2. the new research cluster 'Future of LTC', promoting new technologies in hospital care, residential care and home care.

Germany's 'Digital Strategy'

The 'Digital Strategy' builds upon the 'High-Tech Strategy'; in contrast to the latter, it addresses technology among its key principles on the opening pages where digitisation is presented as a means for improving medical care and for '... facilitating people to live self-determined lives in old age and to enhance their mobility' (BMBF, 2019: 4, authors' translation). Based on these key beliefs, BMBF identifies five target areas in which digitisation and digital change will be implemented, with the first and the fifth explicitly touching upon technology: 1. 'improving quality of life and working conditions in ecologically and economically sustainable ways to improve social participation in rural and urban areas alike by making use of smart applications and services', thereby explicitly referring to smart homes and smart cities; and 5. focusing on digital sovereignty, self-determination and privacy (BMBF, 2019). Under the heading 'We promote digital health innovations for healthcare and LTC', the government's vision for equal access to good-quality healthcare for everybody (urban vs rural, the young vs the old) based on digital innovation is outlined. Several selected research initiatives are presented, including the e-health programme 'Roadmap digital health innovations' (2019–2021), 'Medical computer sciences' programme (2018–2021) or the cluster 'Future of LTC' (since 2015).

More relevant still is the 'implementation strategy of the digital transformation' (Bundesregierung, 2021a, 2021b), which is the result of cross-departmental consultations within the government. The underlying rationale is to scrutinise and, if necessary, readjust the objectives of the strategy. It claims that the overarching objective is to focus more strongly on the intended users. The report is structured in five 'actionable pillars' (Bundesregierung, 2021b):

1. 'Digital competence', integral to digitisation in LTC. Successful funding examples are presented, including: a) the new service point 'digitisation and education for older people'; b) the project 'promoting digital sovereignty of older people with AI technologies'; or c) the new

information platform 'Digital angel' advising older people on digital competencies, such as online banking, using digital services of local authorities and communicating with grandchildren (Bundesregierung, 2021a).

2. 'Infrastructure and equipment' applies to improvements of the telematics infrastructure and IT security in hospital and residential care.
3. 'Innovation and digital transformation', including the application of big data, AI and other new technologies in healthcare but importantly, also the roadmap 'Digital healthcare and LTC' jointly agreed by the departments of Research, Health and Economic Affairs.
4. 'Societal shift toward digitisation'.
5. 'Modern state (governance)'.

Practice

The two sections on 'Principles' and 'Policy' have outlined Germany's strategic position in regard to technology and social care. But how does the implementation of technology work in practice? Families have to organise technology themselves and then ask for reimbursement of related expenses via three mechanisms: 1. LTCI/healthcare insurance; 2. '*Kreditanstalt für Wiederaufbau*' (KfW) loans; and 3. the Digital Provision and LTC Modernisation Act.

Long-term care insurance/healthcare insurance

There are two basic preconditions for being eligible for reimbursement through LTCI: 1. entitlement to LTCI services, that is, a minimum of LTC grade 1; and 2. the requested technology needs to be included in the auxiliary means listings (*Hilfsmittelverzeichnis*). Expenses for very basic auxiliary means are covered by the healthcare insurance provided they are: a) included in their respective auxiliary means listings; and b) they were prescribed by the patient's general practitioner. Whereas health insurance covers the expenses for auxiliary means helping to overcome an illness, LTCI covers expenses for assistive measures in relation to LTC. In practice, it is not always easy to differentiate these subtle differences and care recipients and their families sometimes end up having to submit subsequent reimbursement claims to health insurance and LTCI.

If more substantial 'home environment improving measures' (*wohnumfeldverbessernde Maßnahmen*) are required, people eligible for LTCI can apply for a grant of up to €4,000 from LTCI to make their homes fit for home care and to enable them to continue living independently in their homes. The installation of a smart home could qualify as eligible home improvement, though more common examples include the installation of a stair lift or ground-level showers. If several LTCI recipients cohabit, they are eligible to apply for up to €16,000[1] (BMG, 2021b). However, it is still at the LTCI funds' discretion to reject applications, to pay less than €4,000 and so on – there is no guarantee that applications will be approved. If the care situation changes substantially, a renewed application for another home environment adjustment grant is possible.

Kreditanstalt für Wiederaufbau

The *Kreditanstalt für Wiederaufbau* (KfW) (literal translation 'loan institution for reconstruction') is a so-called *'Förderbank'* (business development bank), that is, a state-owned bank controlled by the Department of Finance of the German government and very unusual by international standards. Judging by its total assets, it is the biggest business development bank in the world, with a balance sheet total of over €500 billion (2020) (KfW, 2020). Even when compared to the private banking sector in Germany, it is third in size after Deutsche Bank and DZ Bank. It is the crucial source of funding for implementing smart home solutions in older people's homes.

KfW offers both grants up to €6,250 and interest-free loans up to €50,000 for home improvements, including the implementation of smart home solutions. This is funded by a specific funding stream, 'Rebuilding age sensitively' (*Altersgerecht umbauen*). If this is combined with energy-efficient reconstruction from a specific energy efficiency promotion programme by central government (*Bundesförderung für effiziente Gebäude*) to make one's home fit for climate change, then grants of up to another €75,000 or interest-free loans of up to €150,000 may be possible (KfW, 2021).

Digital Provision and LTC Modernisation Act

A precondition for any compensation from either health insurance or LTCI is that a medical product or indeed a mobile app is listed in the official list of the Federal Institute for Medication and Medical Products (*Bundesinstitut für Arzneimittel und Medizinprodukte*). In the past, the expenses for mobile health apps could not be reimbursed by health insurance or LTCI since they were not listed in this legally binding list. Until March 2021, 11 new health apps were introduced to this list. According to the umbrella organisation representing all statutory health insurances, some 3,500 digital health apps were prescribed since then (Bundesregierung, 2021a). Another 54 applications to get their mobile apps listed were registered, plus another 450 requests have yet to be dealt with at the time of writing (mid-2022) (Bundesregierung, 2021a).

Similar regulations for the LTC sector were missing until very recently. The German parliament passed the Digital Provision and LTC Modernisation Act (*Digitale-Versorgung-und-Pflege-Modernisierungs-Gesetz*) on 3 June 2021. Care recipients receiving home care are now entitled to digital LTC applications (*digitale Pflegeanwendungen*) and can be reimbursed up to €50 per month (BMG, 2021b). These applications can be used for training and exercises to improve one's health or for improving communication with family carers or professional care workers. Once again, these mobile apps need to be listed in the official list of the Federal Institute for Medication and Medical Products (*Bundesinstitut für Arzneimittel und Medizinprodukte*). This new law allows an accelerated incorporation of digital technologies (care aids, home environment improvements[2]) in LTC and, hence, compensation from LTCI. It was the intention of this law to enable care recipients in home care to take advantage of digital technologies as soon as possible provided that their usefulness is proven. However, this new legislation is still widely unknown and will take time to take effect in practice.

Summary of recent research evidence

The 8th Ageing Report includes a comprehensive state-of-the-art review of relevant publicly available research evidence (Bundestag, 2020). This section will therefore only briefly summarise the findings most relevant to this chapter. Generally speaking, digitisation is framed as major technological revolution embedded in the societal transformation towards an 'information society' (see, for example, Castells, 2001), with both opportunities and risks discussed.

Key to 'digital inclusion' of older people is their competency in using digital devices (Pelizäus-Hoffmeister, 2013). Digital (in)competency is likely to become a new dimension of social inequality, which is referred to as a 'digital divide' (OECD, 2001). Barriers to using digital technologies are far more pronounced among older people than among younger generations. Education, for example, has a much stronger effect, with nearly 90 per cent of well-educated older people using the Internet compared with only 37 per cent of those with low educational attainment (Doh, 2020). If usage of new technologies depends on the availability of financial resources, it aggravates existing social inequality (Künemund, 2016). Although there is no evidence for lower female digital competency in principle, older women are more likely to have worked in low-paid jobs without using digital technology

(Ehlers et al, 2020). Nevertheless, many older people have an overall positive attitude towards digital technology, in particular when they consider it useful. Positive experience in using that technology is crucial for success, which in turn is influenced by usability and data protection (Bundestag, 2020).

From a care worker perspective, digital technologies are often perceived as additional burden or as additional stressor (Institut DGB – Index Gute Arbeit, 2016). Some studies critically reflect the effects of digital documentation systems on daily work routines towards more standardisation and economisation (Hülsken-Giesler 2008; Hergesell 2019). The ambition by (some) employers to substitute the work of care assistants by digital means is often seen as cause for concern. It has been suggested that up to half of all auxiliary care services could be digitised in future (Bundestag, 2020). However, the vast majority of care experts agree on a complementary role for digital devices and services. Digital substitution of human care work is seen as morally unjustified since it infringes on the self-determination of care recipients (Bundestag, 2020). Moreover, there is little reliable evidence on greater efficiency of digital devices in LTC since existing studies are based on small samples or have methodological limitations (Bundestag, 2020). Furthermore, there is no empirical evidence for health-related utility of telecare applications (Klein and Oswald, 2020). The 8th Ageing Report concludes that it remains to be seen if this position will hold against a background of dynamic technology development and continued labour shortages in the care market, which have been aggravated by the COVID-19 pandemic (Bundestag, 2020).

Conclusion

LTC is among the least glamorous professional domains in Germany. The COVID-19 pandemic focused public attention on LTC, making visible growing deficiencies due to decades of underfunding and care worker shortages. Changes in family norms (female labour market participation, responsibility for caregiving) and family structures (fewer children, increasing geographical distance between the generations) challenge the sustainability of previous informal care arrangements. LTC highlights the enormous tensions German society is facing, which have remained unsolved for too long.

Technology could help to solve the conundrum by enabling older people to live independently in their homes longer and by enabling so-called 'distance caregiving' (Franke et al, 2019). However, precondition is reliable and fast Internet all across the country and not just metropolitan areas. A clear vision and a realistic strategy of how to implement technology in LTC are missing. Moreover, the lack of leadership and coordination at central government level (research department vs health department) and the enormous time lag between technology development and their inclusion into legislation governing LTC are major obstacles for a more widespread use of assistive technologies in home care. While there is a variety of research programmes for technology development based on the latest technological advances, potential users find it hard to get reliable information and advice on technology, on how to get them installed in their homes and from which sources to get financial support. As a consequence, there is limited awareness and use of technology in caring contexts by older people and their families. Many find it difficult to get reimbursed for using technology from LTCI. It remains to be seen if the 2021 Digital Provision and LTC Modernisation Act will change that as people become aware of this new legislation.

Furthermore, the vast majority of state-of-the-art technology developed in research programmes never makes it to marketisation. The result is an enormous waste of creativity and money. Technological advances do not take into consideration the needs and preferences of the intended user group. In our opinion, participative technology development, that is, co-creation of technology by engineers and scientists with older people and informal/formal caregivers working as equal partners, would be a sensible way forward to make sure that people get technologies they really want (see Weidner and Redlich, 2014). Moreover, older people and their carers should be empowered to make their own judgements on the risks associated with using technologies rather than relying on the risk analysis by developers or care providers. Such 'digital empowerment' of technology users is most likely to be sustainable given the rapid development of new devices and systems.

Notes

1 One person can apply for up to €4,000, two for up to €8,000, three for up to €12,000, and four and more people for up to €16,000.

2 In German: *Pflegehilfsmittel und wohnumfeldverbessernde Maßnahmen*.

References

Althammer, J., Lampert, H. and Sommer, M. (2021) *Lehrbuch der Sozialpolitik* (10th edition). Heidelberg: Springer Gabler Berlin.

Anttonen, A. and Sipilä, J. (1996) 'European social care services: is it possible to identify models?', *Journal of European Social Policy*, 6(2): 87–100.

Bundesagentur für Arbeit. (2021) 'Arbeitsmarktsituation im pflegebereich', Blickpunkt Arbeitsbereich. Available at: https://statistik.arbeitsagentur.de/DE/Statischer-Content/Statistiken/Themen-im-Fokus/Berufe/Generische-Publikationen/Altenpflege.pdf?__blob=publicationFile&v=13#:~:text=Im%20Jahr%202021%20hat%20es%20keine%20merkliche%20Ver%C3%A4nderung%20der%20Arbeitslosenzahl%20gegeben.&text=Die%20Zahl%20der%20gemeldeten%20Stellen,%C3%BCbersteigt%20die%20der%20Arbeitslosen%20deutlich [accessed 25.11.22].

Bundesinstitut für Bevölkerungsforschung [BiB]. (2021) 'Demografiestrategie der bundesregierung'. Available at: https://www.demografie-portal.de/DE/Politik/Bund/demografiestrategie.html [accessed 25.11.22].

Bundesministerium für Bildung und Forschung [BMBF]. (2013) 'Themen im Wissenschaftsjahr 2013'. Die Demographische Chance. Available at: https://www.demografie-portal.de/DE/Service/Blog/130130-wissenschaftsjahr-2013-demografische-chance.html [accessed 25.11.22].

Bundesministerium für Bildung und Forschung. (2018a) 'Forschung und Innovation für die Menschen. Die Hightech-Strategie 2025'. Available at: https://www.bundesgesundheitsministerium.de/fileadmin/Dateien/3_Downloads/B/BuFI/Bundesbericht_Forschung_und_Innovation_2018_barrierefrei.pdf [accessed 25.11.22].

Bundesministerium für Bildung und Forschung. (2018b) 'Research and innovation that benefit the people. The High-Tech Strategy 2025'. Available at: https://www.bundesregierung.de/breg-en/service/archive/report-high-tech-strategy-1930002 [accessed 25.11.22].

Bundesministerium für Bildung und Forschung. (2019) 'Digitale Zukunft: Lernen. Forschen. Wissen. Die Digitalstrategie des BMBF'. Available at https://www.bildung-forschung.digital/digitalezukunft/shareddocs/Downloads/files/bmbf_digitalstrategie.pdf [accessed 25.11.22].

Bundesministerium für Bildung und Forschung. (2021) 'Bericht der bundesregierung zur hightech-strategie 2025. Erfolgsmodell hightech-strategie für ein starkes Innovationsland Deutschland'. Available at: https://www.bmbf.de/SharedDocs/Publikationen/de/bmbf/1/138398_Bericht_zur_Hightech-Strategie_2025.pdf?__blob=publicationFile&v=5 [accessed 25.11.22].

Bundesministerium für Familie, Senioren, Frauen und Jugend [BMFSFJ]. (2021) 'Reconciliation of family, care and work'. Available at: https://www.bmfsfj.de/bmfsfj/meta/en/senior-citizens [accessed 25.11.22].

Bundesministerium für Gesundheit [BMG]. (2021a) 'Zahlen und Fakten zur Pflegeversicherung'. Available at: https://www.bundesgesundheitsministerium.de/themen/pflege/pflegeversicherung-zahlen-und-fakten.html [accessed 25.11.22].

Bundesministerium für Gesundheit. (2021b) 'Wohnumfeldverbessernde maßnahmen' Available at: https://www.bundesgesundheitsministerium.de/leistungen-der-pflege/wohnumfeldverbessernde-massnahmen.html [accessed 25.11.22].

Bundesministerium für Gesundheit. (2022) 'Vereinbarkeit von pflege und beruf'. Available at: https://www.bundesgesundheitsministerium.de/leistungen-der-pflege/vereinbarkeit-von-pflege-und-beruf.html [accessed 29.11.22].

Bundesregierung. (2021a) 'Digitalisierung gestalten. Die Umsetzungsstrategie der Bundesregierung 6'. Available at: https://www.bundesregierung.de/resource/blob/992814/1605036/339a38c264fd50ff9efca6ad8da64bae/digitalisierung-gestalten-download-bpa-data.pdf?download=1 [accessed 25.11.22].

Bundesregierung. (2021b) 'Shaping digitisation: implementation strategy of the Federal Government'. Available at: https://www.bundesregierung.de/resource/blob/992814/1605342/284988700922725d63a0fb95db824024/digitalsierung-gestalten-englisch-download-bpa-data.pdf?download=1 [accessed 25.11.22].

Bundestag. (1994) *Elftes Buch Sozialgesetzbuch Soziale Pflegeverischerung,* Berlin: Bundestag.

Bundestag. (2020). *Gesetz für eine bessere Versorgung durch Digitalisierung und Innovation (Digitale-Versorgung-Gesetz – DVG),* Berlin: Bundestag.

Castells, M. (2001) *Der Aufstieg der Netzwerkgesellschaft. Teil I der Trilogie Das Informationszeitalter,* New York: Leske and Budrich.

Destatis. (2020) 'Pflegestatistik - Pflege im Rahmen der Pflegeversicherung - Deutschlandergebnisse – 2019'. Available at: https://www.destatis.de/DE/Themen/Gesellschaft-Umwelt/Gesundheit/Pflege/Publikationen/Downloads-Pflege/pflege-deutschlandergebnisse-5224001199004.html [accessed 25.11.22].

Doh, M. (2020) 'Auswertung von empirischen Studien zur Nutzung von Internet, digitalen Medien und Informations- und Kommunikations-Technologien bei älteren Menschen'. Expertise zum Achten Altersbericht der Bundesregierung, Issue. Available at: https://www.achter-altersbericht.de/fileadmin/altersbericht/pdf/Expertisen/Expertise-Doh.pdf [accesssed 24.01.23].

Ehlers, A., Heß, M., Frewer-Graumann, S. and Olbermann, E. (2020) 'Digitale Teilhabe und (digitale) Exklusion im Alter'. Expertise zum Achten Altersbericht der Bundesregierung, Issue. Geschäftsstelle für die Altersberichte der Bundesregierung, Deutsches Zentrum für Altersfragen

Engstler, H. and Tesch-Römer, C. (2017) 'Zeitverwendung von Erwachsenen, die ein Haushaltsmitglied pflegen'. *Wie die Zeit vergeht: Analysen zur Zeitverwendung 2012/2013 in Deutschland. Beiträge zur Ergebniskonferenz der Zeitverwendungserhebung 2012/2013*. Berlin: Statistisches Bundesamt.

Esping-Andersen, G. (1990). *The Three Worlds of Welfare Capitalism*. Princeton, New Jersey: Princeton University Press.

European Commission [EC]. (2021) 'Long-term care report. Trends, challenges and opportunities in an ageing society (Vol. 2)', Luxembourg: Publications Office of the European Union.

Eurostat. (2020) 'Anteil der Bevölkerung ab 65 Jahren in Ländern Europas 2019'. Available at: https://de.statista.com/statistik/daten/studie/243939/umfrage/anteil-der-bevoelkerung-ab-65-in-laendern-europas/ [accessed 25.11.22].

Franke, A., Kramer, B., Jann, P.M., van Holten, K., Zentgraf, A., Otto, U., et al (2019) 'Aktuelle Befunde zu 'distance caregiving', *Zeitschrift für Gerontologie und Geriatrie*, 52(6): 521–528.

Geyer, J. (2016) 'Informell Pflegende in der deutschen Erwerbsbevölkerung: Soziodemografie, Pflegesituation und Erwerbsverhalten'. *Themenreport: Vereinbarkeit von Beruf und Pflege*, Berlin: ZQP, pp 24–43.

Hayek, A., Lehnert, T., Wegener, A., Riedel-Heller, S. and König, H.-H. (2018) 'Langzeitpräferenzen der Älteren in Deutschland. Ergebnisse einer bevölkerungsrepräsentativen Umfrage', *Gesundheitswesen*, 80(08–09): 685–692.

Hergesell, J. (2019) 'Von der Armen-und Siechenfürsorge zur digitalisierten Altenpflege. Eine figurationssoziologische Perspektive auf Pflegeinnovationen' in Ernst, S. and Becke, G. (Eds) *Transformationen der Arbeitsgesellschaft*, Wiesbaden: Springer VS, pp 235–258.

Hielscher, V., Kirchen-Peters, S. and Nock, L. (2017) *Pflege in den eigenen vier Wänden: Zeitaufwand und Kosten*, (No. 363). Stuttgart, Germany: Study der Hans-Böckler-Stiftung.

Hülsken-Giesler, M. (2008) 'Self-directed learning with new media – care (from) education between personality development and educational technology', *bwp@*, special, 4: 1–6.

Institut DGB – Index Gute Arbeit (2016) *Schwerpunkt: Digitalisierung der Arbeitswelt.*

Institut-DGB-Index-Gute-Arbeit. (2018). *Report 2016 - Schwerpunkt: digitalisierung der arbeitswelt.* Available at: https://index-gute-arbeit.dgb.de/veroeffentlichungen/kompakt/++co++bf2674ba-0a6a-11e8-bcc4-52540088cada [accessed 25.11.22].

Jacobs, K., Kuhlmey, A., Greß, S., Klauber, J. and Schwinger, A. (Eds). (2021) *Pflege-Report 2021: Sicherstellung der Pflege: Bedarfslagen und Angebotsstrukturen*, New York: Springer.

Klein, B. and Oswald, F. (2020) 'Möglichkeiten und Herausforderungen der Implementierung von Technologien' in Herausgegeben von C. Hagen, C. Endter und F. Berner (Eds) *Alltag von älteren Menschen: Expertise zum Achten Altersbericht der Bundesre-gierung*, Berlin: Deutsches Zentrum für Altersfragen.

Kreditanstalt für Wiederaufbau [KfW]. (2020) 'Financial report 2020', Frankfurt, Germany: KfW. Available at: https://www.kfw.de/PDF/Download-Center/Finanzpublikationen/PDF-Dokumente-Berichte-etc/3_Finanzberichte/Finanzbericht_2020-2.pdf [accessed 22.02.23].

Kreditanstalt für Wiederaufbau. (2021) 'Ihr smart home – intelligent gesteuert und staatlich gefördert'. Available at: https://www.kfw.de/inlandsfoerderung/Privatpersonen/Bestandsimmobilie/Smart-Home/ [accessed 25.11.22].

Kuhlmey, A., Dräger, D. and Winter, M. (2010) 'COMPASS – Versichertenbefragung zu Erwartungen und Wünschen an eine qualitativ gute Pflege', *Informationsdienst Altersfragen*, 37(4): 4–11.

Künemund, H. (2016) 'Wovon hängt die Nutzung technischer Assistenzsysteme ab? Expertise zum Siebten Altenbericht der Bundesregierung', Berlin. Available at: https://www.siebter-altenbericht.de/fileadmin/altenbericht/pdf/Expertise_Kuenemund.pdf [accessed 22.02.23].

OECD. (2001) 'Understanding the Digital Divide', Paris: OECD. Available at: https://www.oecd-ilibrary.org/science-and-technology/understanding-the-digital-divide_236405667766 [accessed 21.02.23].

Pelizäus-Hoffmeister, H. (2013) *Zur Bedeutung von Technik im Alltag Älterer: Theorie und Empirie aus soziologischer Perspektive* (Vol. 24), New York: Springer-Verlag.

Rothgang, H., Müller, R. and Preuß, B. (2020) 'BARMER Pflegereport 2020: Belastungen der Pflegekräfte und ihre Folgen', Berlin: BARMER. Available at: https://www.socium.uni-bremen.de/uploads/News/2020/20201201_BARMER_Pflegereport_2020.pdf [accessed 21.02.23].

Statista (2020) 'Number of people in private long-term care in Germany from 1997–2019'. Available at: https://de.statista.com/statistik/daten/studie/6676/umfrage/private-pflegeversicherung-anzahl-der-versicherten-seit-1997/ [accessed 25.11.22].

Unabhängiger-Beirat-Vereinbarkeit-Pflege-Beruf. (2019) 'Erster Bericht des unabhängigen Beirats für die Vereinbarkeit von Pflege und Beruf'. Available at: https://www.wege-zur-pflege.de/fileadmin/daten/Beirat/Erster_Bericht_des_unabhaengigen_Beirats_2019.pdf [accessed 25.11.22].

Weidner, R. and Redlich, T. (Eds). (2014) *Technische Unterstützungssysteme, die die Menschen wirklich wollen*, Hamburg: Helmut-Schmidt-University Press.

FIVE

Technology and care in Canada

Arlene Astell and Janet Fast

Social care: policy, debates and evidence

Structure of social care

Canada's population of 38,526,760 people (Statistics Canada, 2022) is spread across 3,855,103 square miles in the second largest country in the world. The country comprises ten provinces and three territories, which share power with the federal government. Each province and territory elects its own government to create laws on public education, health and social services. The geography of the country and the distribution of centres of population contribute to a unique landscape in which care at home is delivered.

Against this backdrop, Canada has no national social care 'system' per se. The Canada Health Act, adopted in 1984, is federal legislation that established criteria and conditions for insured healthcare services and extended healthcare services, which the provinces and territories must provide to receive the full Canada Health Transfer (CHT). CHT is a federal cash contribution to the cost of providing health services (delivery of which is the responsibility of the provinces and territories).

The primary objective of the Canada Health Act is 'to protect, promote and restore the physical and mental well-being of residents of Canada and to facilitate reasonable access to health services without financial or other barriers.' Insured services include medically necessary in-patient and out-patient hospital services and medically required physician services. That is, the Act does not require provinces to provide social care supports and services.

Social care services are nevertheless provided in Canada, both by the provinces and territories and by the federal government to specific populations, including Aboriginal and Inuit peoples, Armed Forces personnel, federal inmates and eligible veterans. 'Home and community care services', as these are called in Canada, help people receive care at home, rather than in a hospital or Long-Term Care (LTC) facility, and to live as independently as possible in the community.

The Conference Board of Canada's conceptual framework (Hermus et al, 2012) for home and community care comprises four core domains: 1. 'Home health and support services'; 2. 'Community care services'; 3. 'Voluntary donations and services'; and 4. 'Family caregiving'. In Canada, home care programmes include personal care alongside professional health services (for example, nursing, physiotherapy, occupational therapy, social work), plus case management. Community care services typically complement home care services and may include meal preparation, homemaking, palliative care, 'meals on wheels' (delivery of hot or 'heat and serve' meals), friendly visitors, transportation, community dining, mental healthcare and supportive housing. Integration of community care with other services varies across provinces (Lukey et al, 2021).

Funding

Home care in Canada is funded both publicly and privately and delivered by for-profit and not-for-profit service providers

(CIHI, 2010). Publicly funded clients receive care in one of two ways: through a contracted agency paid for by the relevant government; or through a home care agency paid for by a client who receives a monthly stipend from the government to 'shop' for home care that best meets their needs (sometimes referred to as 'self-managed care'). Public funding comes from the federal government by way of the CHT and from general provincial tax revenues. Bilateral funding agreements negotiated in the late 2010s between the national government in Ottawa and the provincial governments included additional funds for making improvements to home care services (Johnson et al, 2017). However, public funding covers only a portion of the costs for only a portion of users. Access to publicly funded home and community care is means-tested in all jurisdictions. In addition, there is typically a cap on the amount of subsidy provided, including to eligible users. If the service provider's fee exceeds the provincial cap, the user must make up the difference. Users whose earnings exceed the provincial cap must pay the full fee charged by the service provider. The share of costs borne by the client and by government varies by province.

Eligibility

Eligibility for home care is assessed by a case manager or through other professional assessment. Basic eligibility to receive services includes status as a Canadian citizen or Permanent Resident or holding a Temporary Resident permit – these are required to receive a Health Card. A period of residence in the relevant province, commonly three months, is typically but not always expected. Across the country, home care services are available for individuals who have functional limitations due to chronic or life-limiting health conditions that require care. Eligibility for cost subsidies is based on income. Some services are free to eligible residents, while others, such as those described as 'homemaking' may require a financial contribution (Johnson et al, 2017).

The ten Canadian provinces differ in their eligibility criteria for subsidies. In British Columbia, home care is available to residents who 'have been assessed as requiring personal assistance and/or respite for your caregiver through a clinical assessment by a health authority health care professional; and have agreed to pay the assessed client rate' (British Columbia Government, 2022). In Saskatchewan, residents can apply for 'individualised funding' to arrange, manage and report their own support services, which includes recruitment, hiring, training and termination of staff (Saskatchewan.ca, n.d.). A similar system of self-managed care operates in Nova Scotia, Manitoba and Ontario, which also offer 'family-managed care'. In Quebec, there is a tax credit for expenses relating to home care services, including nursing care, housekeeping and meal preparation. This is available for residents over 70 years of age based on criteria that include place of residence and family income. Similarly, in Alberta, income status and smoking status are assessed as part of the eligibility process. In Prince Edward Island, Community Support and Home Support services require residence plus a means test and a needs test (Health PEI, 2022). The New Brunswick Long Term Care Program provides home care assistance, including getting dressed, bathing, cooking and managing medication. To qualify, individuals must be aged 65 years or older; live in New Brunswick; consent to a functional assessment (of personal care and social needs); be medically stable (not receiving care and treatment that will significantly improve their condition); have limited ability to do daily activities and have personal care needs not met by someone else; require services on a long-term basis; and consent to financial assessment (Social Supports NB, 2022). In Labrador and Newfoundland, the Provincial Home Support Program includes a means and needs assessment and a residence requirement plus a Paid Family Caregiving Option, where a family member can receive the subsidy to provide care in lieu of services.

The three Canadian territories (Northwest Territories, Yukon and Nunavut) are collectively home to approximately

118,160 people, roughly 0.3 per cent of the total population. They live in 1,349,922 square miles, or roughly 35 per cent of Canada's landmass. The vastness of these northern territories and the smallness of the populations present challenges for home care delivery. In 2017, the governments of these territories agreed with the federal government a CAD$36.1 million funding package that included $19.7 million for home care infrastructure (Government of Canada, 2017). However, a 2019 consultation in the Northwest Territories identified a major problem with lack of awareness and confusion regarding eligibility for home care services (Government of the Northwest Territories, 2020). To improve communication, flyers were produced to inform communities that 'anyone residing in the Territory who has a valid NWT health card is eligible' (NTHSSA, 2022). Similarly in Nunavut, anyone enrolled in the Nunavut Health Care Plan is eligible for referral to the Home and Community Care programme (Nunavut Government, 2022). In Yukon, residents of all ages with an assessed need for home care and a Yukon Health Care Insurance Plan are eligible for home care (Yukon.ca, 2022).

The role of family and friend carers

As in many of the other countries included in this book, most care in Canada is provided by family/friend carers. Indeed, as Hermus et al (2012) observed, many researchers and advocates have observed that the health system would be unable to cope without the unpaid labour provided by family, friends and community members or volunteers. In 2018, approximately 25 per cent of all Canadians over 15 years of age (7.8 million people) provided care to at least one family member or friend with long-term physical or mental health conditions, disabilities or age-related conditions (Statistics Canada, 2020). For many formal home and community care providers, availability of a primary family carer is a condition for receipt of services. Eales et al (2022) reported that in 2018, Canadian family carers spent

5.7 billion hours on care tasks annually, the monetary value of which they estimated as equal to 37 per cent of all public healthcare spending and three times national expenditures on home, community and LTC in the same year.

Social care: key statistics

In 2015/2016, 6.4 per cent of Canadian households (881,800) reported that at least one person had received formal home care services in the previous 12 months (Gilmour, 2018). Total health spending in Canada is expected to reach CAD$308 billion in 2021, or CAD$8,019 per Canadian, representing 12.7 per cent of Canada's gross domestic product. In 2020–21, home and continuing care accounted for just over 5 per cent of total provincial healthcare spending, while another 11 per cent went towards residential LTC. By comparison, about 25 per cent of all healthcare expenditures was allocated to hospitals (Busby, 2021).

Numerous reports published in recent years, including the Romanow report (2002), Kirby report (2002) and 'Bringing Care Home' report (Ontario Government, 2015), have called for improvements across all jurisdictions to home and community care services. Recommendations have included increased funding, more stringent service delivery standards and amending the Canada Health Act to include home and community care among the mandated healthcare services. Gilmore (2018) reported that in 2015/16, over one third of people with home care needs did not have those needs met, with lack of available services identified as the most common barrier to obtaining home care services. Those with complex care needs were at greatest risk of not receiving the full scope of care that they needed.

Social care and technology: research, practice and policy

Technology and care policy and practice

While provinces are responsible for delivery of home and community care services, including care technologies, the federal government plays an important regulatory role regarding healthcare technologies. Under current legislation, care recipients can access technology and digital services through means-tested processes. The types of technologies typically available include emergency response systems, such as medical alerts and remote monitoring. Medical alert systems include Lifeline (New Brunswick) and MedicAlert (Saskatchewan); in Alberta, clients who qualify can receive benefits to cover the cost of a medical alert system of their choice.

Interestingly, both New Brunswick and British Columbia offer access to remote monitoring systems that support unpaid carers. New Brunswick offers CareLink Advantage (Social Supports NB, 2022) while British Columbia has a partnership with telecoms provider TELUS for home health monitoring. CareLink Advantage is presented as a 'passive' system for the care recipient, which includes door and bed sensors to track their movements at home. TELUS Home Health monitoring has been in place in British Columbia since 2013.

In most parts of Canada, with the exception of Labrador and Newfoundland (see 'Eligibility' above), family carers cannot currently access province-funded technologies to support their roles. With the lack of a business-to-business chain whereby technology companies sell to healthcare or home care providers, there is less incentive for companies to develop digital tools for family carers. As such, there is currently little focus on technology development for carers and consequently scant awareness of their needs. With almost half the adult population of Canada providing some form of care, there is nevertheless clearly both a huge need and a potential market.

There has been federal investment in research and development in care and technology, notably through the establishment of AGE-WELL in 2015 (through Canada's Networks of Centres of Excellence programme), which aimed to stimulate and promote the development and adoption of products and services to support people to age well in Canada. AGE-WELL recognises the massive contribution of families to caring for their older members and their need for digital resources. It is also concerned with contributing to policy change to increase equity of access to, and the availability of, digital supports for Canada's ageing population. In 2017, AGE-WELL established a National Innovation Hub, 'APPTA', to lead policy innovation. It is also increasing awareness and stimulating creation of technologies to support caring. Achieving this requires promotion of caring as a market. One AGE-WELL partner, the electronics retailer Best Buy, has recognised this and now offers a range of products to support caring.

With care technology still in its infancy in Canada, current development efforts are primarily led by companies rather than provinces. They fall into four main domains: 1. care management/coordination; 2. smart homes; 3. outdoor tracking; and 4. communication technologies.

1: Care management and coordination

Most digital resources for care management and coordination are aimed at home care companies rather than family or other unpaid carers. While numerous companies care for individuals in their own homes, most do not connect with family carers. An exception is Servus Health, a platform for matching older adults and families with care providers, a finalist in AGE-WELL's 2020 National Impact Challenge. FamliNet, an AGE-WELL–supported start-up company, is another app developed in Canada that aims to support some aspects of care management and coordination. The FamliNet tools include an app and step-by-step instructions to engage older adults with digital activities and support them to connect online. It is based on prior research by its founder into how older adults learn to use digital tools (Leone et al, 2018). FamliNet promotes digital engagement to give family carers a break and has the functionality to create a family circle to support communication within families. Testimonials on its website present user stories, including those of family carers and the benefits they experience from using FamliNet. Other companies offering smart home sensing and monitoring also include an app or other interface for family carers.

Another company seeking to reduce demands on family carers by supporting older adults at home is Custodia, which provides helpers for 'companionship, home maintenance, gardening/yard work, odd jobs and assistance with household tasks'. Registration is free; older adults seeking assistance are matched with helpers in their local community and jobs are charged per task. Custodia offers a technology-based service with all booking completed online and aiming to support older adults to stay in their homes longer. Its founder noticed his mother struggling to keep on top of home maintenance tasks and felt that resolving these could make it possible for her to continue living in her home. Between its establishment in 2019 and the end of 2020, Custodia's website reports booking over 17,000 service visits. The company also partners with other home care providers in communities across Ontario and two communities in British Columbia. No research evidence is available on this matching service, but figures for numbers of visits booked suggest a desire and need for the service. The model of linking older adults with helpers in their local community is potentially scalable across Canada and beyond.

2: Smart homes

The potential of sensors in homes to monitor various aspects of a resident's health and behaviour is increasingly being explored. The data generated can be shared with family carers to help them manage care and provide reassurance regarding their spouse or parent's well-being, particularly if they are at work or are not co-resident. In Ottawa, the Sensors and Analytics for Monitoring Mobility and Memory (SAM3) AGE-WELL Innovation Hub is investigating a range of sensors to support ageing well. Its projects for carers have demonstrated results for its Night-time Wandering Detection and Diversion system for people living with dementia that include a reduction in depression and improved sleep (Ault et al, 2020). Another ongoing project is assessing use of sensor data to detect changes in caring activities, with the aim of providing targeted feedback to reduce carer stress (Ault et al, 2020; Thomas et al, 2020). While an area of emerging interest among developers and people who draw on care and support, most provinces do not support smart home technologies, with the exception of British Columbia and New Brunswick where remote monitoring is available (as already described).

Commercial smart home products are also becoming more popular. Five of the 15 finalists in the AGE-WELL 2020 National Impact Challenge were companies using sensors and smart devices: HomeEXCEPT, eNable Analytics, Novalte and Tochtech Technologies. Three of these – eNable Analytics, Novalte and Tochtech – won their regional finals. Best Buy, another AGE-WELL partner, is both a supplier of smart home technology and collaborator on smart home projects, including the SAM3 innovation hub.

3: Tracking

A major initiative within AGE-WELL has been keeping people living with dementia safe when they go out, and reassuring family carers that they are safe. Work by researchers in Ontario and Alberta has established the acceptability of GPS devices and the benefits they can bring to family dyads (Liu et al, 2017). In addition, the interdisciplinary team was involved in work to amend Canada's Missing Person's Act, which allowed police to obtain access to a missing person's information with the aim of introducing a 'Silver Alert' across Canada (a public announcement made when a person with dementia goes missing). This has yet to be adopted across Canada, but Vancouver has a citizen-funded Silver Alert programme, and in Manitoba, legislation is under consideration to enable use of provincial funding for the programme. First established in the US, the Silver Alert has been emulated in other countries, including Scotland's Purple Alert.

4: Communications technologies

AGE-WELL researchers examining caring have explored the mediating role technology plays in accessing information and support, finding that digital support is crucial for carers in rural and remote parts of Canada. Two new projects funded by the Saskatchewan Health Research Foundation are examining how the Internet can be used to deliver culturally safe support to carers of people living with dementia in indigenous communities. The first, led by Saskatchewan's Rural and Remote Memory Clinic and the University of Saskatchewan, is examining the impact of monthly support group sessions accessed online to explore whether these help family carers manage stress. The second, led by researchers from the Morning Star Lodge indigenous community-based lab in Regina, provides family carers with tablets and Internet connectivity to access tailored information and resources. This builds on AGE-WELL work on the use of apps to reduce carer stress in indigenous communities (Starblanket and Legare, 2019; Starblanket et al, 2019).

Summary of recent research evidence

In 2009, Alberta Health and Wellness (in partnership with Alberta Health Services) commissioned the 'Continuing Care Health Technologies Roadmap' (InnoTraction Solutions Inc., 2009) as part of its strategy to support ageing in place. The roadmap comprised five areas – global review, current state assessment, technology roadmap, technology recommendations and implementation considerations – with the aim of assessing current availability and identifying emerging technologies. In line with studies across Canada, the roadmap identified 'telehealth' and 'telecare' as key areas. This reflects in part the size and distribution of the population in Canada, where digital services for people in rural and remote areas are essential. Despite this, Owens (2018) found that Canada was behind other countries in adopting telemedicine and virtual consultations. The subsequent COVID-19 pandemic has stimulated upscaling of virtual health and care delivery, as in many other countries. Kaminski (2021) highlights telehealth as delivering three key benefits: 1. improved access to care (subject to the technology being available – a substantial caveat); 2. promoting continuity of care, particularly for individuals living with multiple long-term conditions; and 3. improved resource use, including physician time.

A 2022 review focusing on the needs of older Canadians identified the need for specific 'virtual care-related policies' to ensure older adults are not left behind; action to address limited uptake of virtual care by disadvantaged communities; and the promotion of person-centred design and iterative evaluation processes for new devices and services (Pang et al, 2022). The review findings accord with concerns raised by older people in British Columbia and California living with multiple chronic conditions about the rise of 'surveillance technologies' as part of home care systems, alongside some potential benefits (Mortensonet al, 2016). Others have reported a lack of evidence for technology-based interventions relative to interventions delivered at home by healthcare professionals (Welch et al, 2021).

While the main focus in policy and by developers has been on care technologies for populations in need of care at home, the development of digital resources for unpaid carers is also attracting attention. A growing number of projects are developing technologies, and companies such as HomeEXCEPT are offering technology to support care at home. AGE-WELL has supported Huddol, a platform run by the Canadian Caregiver Network, to add artificial intelligence as part of its work to create devices, services and policies for carers, and has hosted various initiatives to explore and capture the needs of family carers, current gaps and problems in caring technology and to raise awareness of these needs. A dedicated Caregiving YouTube channel provides stories that illustrate different care trajectories, complemented by an AGE-WELL tool for crowdsourcing carer personas, aimed at technology developers, clinicians and other caregivers, to identify existing and novel solutions. The personas are created through a survey of caregivers. A further AGE-WELL tool (CARE-RATE) uses natural language processing where computers are programmed to analyse speech to enable family carers to describe a specific problem they are experiencing. Cognitive computing allows CARE-RATE to offer the carer suggestions about assistive technology, online resources, forums and strategies that can help.

To explore the challenges family carers face, AGE-WELL's DATcares team identified seven barriers to adopting technology (Eales et al, 2017):

1. lack of information about available technology and how to access it;
2. failure of existing technology to solve carers' problems;
3. affordability of existing technology and need to self-pay;
4. lack of Internet access;
5. lack of support for using digital tools;
6. inadequate digital skills; and
7. impact of technology on caring relationships.

The second barrier – the failure of existing technology to meet the carers' needs – could be addressed through greater engagement between technology researchers, producers and suppliers, family carers and older adults needing care. To increase engagement, AGE-WELL has over 200 partner organisations, including more than 60 industrial partners, and runs regular interaction workshops and activities to bring these groups together.

Another support is the CareDATA tool, created specifically to support technology developers to engage with family carers, identify their needs and preferences, break down barriers to technology adoption and enhance uptake. Developed through interviews with carers, technology developers and researchers (Xiong et al, 2022), CareDATA is a freely available resource with guidance on how to engage and work together. As it is funded by the Canadian Institutes of Health Research Sex and Gender-Based Analysis Policy-Research Partnerships, CareDATA provides guidance for incorporating sex, gender and other forms of diversity in developing caring technology, based on research on the needs of diverse family carers (Xiong et al, 2018; Xiong et al, 2020). Its use in promoting greater use of co-production and improved recognition of diverse carer needs is currently under evaluation.

In addition to encouraging dialogue and co-production between technology developers, carers and care recipients, there is also a need for more caring technology projects and partnerships that go beyond pilot or feasibility stage to become commercial products or services. This, as already indicated, arises partly from perceptions about the market for caring technology and the lack of expressed demand by major business customers, such as healthcare or home care providers, for these products. There is nevertheless a strong business case in the direct impact caring has on employers. In Canada, family care responsibilities are estimated to result in 9.7 million days of absenteeism, 256 million fewer hours of paid work, and the loss of 557,698 caregiver employees who left the paid labour force altogether to provide care (Fast et al, 2014). Promoting development of caring technologies to empower employees to remain in employment while providing care is thus an important priority.

As part of its mission to develop policy, AGE-WELL's Assistive Technologies that Care for the Caregiver (AtforCC) project examined carers' needs and goals and how assistive technology could impact their lives. Data were collected from a survey and focus groups, finding that carers identified technology as a potential support in developing their resilience to continue caring. Barriers identified included limited availability and functionality for connecting carers to online resources such as peer or social support and information. Findings are being used to inform: evidence-based policy decisions, non-governmental organisation advocacy efforts and development and adoption of AGE-WELL products (Leslie et al, 2020).

Conclusion

Social care is not a public policy category in Canada in the same way as in some other countries discussed in this book. Responsibility for the organisation and delivery of care at home is devolved to Canada's provinces and territories, resulting in considerable variability in services and support across the country. The availability of technology and eligibility for publicly funded support vary according to means, and in most of Canada, carers have no access to government funding for technology to support them in their caring role.

As in some other countries, the COVID-19 pandemic accelerated the move to virtual and remote service delivery. In 2020, a Deloitte report proclaimed 'COVID-19: Virtual care is here to stay', observing that 'for Canada to have a sustainable health care system, virtual care must become a permanent outcome of the COVID-19 pandemic' (Deloitte, 2020: 1) and identifying multiple benefits to the healthcare system, including improved care quality and coordination; increased efficiency and decreased costs; enhanced clinical outcomes and experience for users; and improved accessibility of care with reduced geographical disparities. Telehealth and remote monitoring are highlighted as technologies to enhance resource utilisation and patient self-management, as are the cost benefits to the healthcare system of virtual care (estimated at more than CAN$30 billion in benefits accrued since 2017). Interestingly, there is no mention of the critical role that family and other informal carers play in maintaining people at home or how technology can alleviate the pressure on them.

However, Canada is a vast country, and its many people living in rural and remote areas are extremely disadvantaged in terms of Internet connectivity. Two government initiatives,

Canada's Connectivity Strategy (Innovation, Science and Economic Development Canada, 2019a) and Rural Economic Development Strategy (Innovation, Science and Economic Development Canada, 2019b), were introduced to provide Internet and device access to vulnerable and socio-economically disadvantaged individuals, families and communities. Meanwhile, telehealth and telecare are growing rapidly with more than 353,000 people accessing 'virtual care' in 2021 (Ontario Telemedicine Network, 2023).

Canada's national ageing and technology network AGE-WELL was established in 2015 and implemented 11 projects to explore technology for family caring in its first five years, covering topics ranging from providing advice to carers about technology acquisition to assistive technologies to care for the carer. It has also produced position papers and a national hub dedicated to influencing policy on technology in relation to ageing. Technology to support caring is on the increase in Canada but evidence about the efficacy and impact of these systems and devices is not yet available, with systems still in their infancy and long-term data (for example, on reducing demands on carers or the need to give up paid work to provide care, and on improving carers' physical and mental well-being) not yet available.

References

Ault, L., Goubran, R., Wallace, B., Lowden, H. and Knoefel, F. (2020) 'Smart home technology solution for night-time wandering in persons with dementia', *Journal of Rehabilitation and Assistive Technologies Engineering*, 7: doi:10.1177/2055668320938591.

Ault, L., Kachala, A., Knoefel, F., Frank, A., Wallace, B., Kaye, J., et al (2020) 'Developing a caregiver feedback response system using a home-based sensor platform', *Gerontechnology*, 19(0): 1–1.

British Columbia Government. (2022) 'Home and community care'. Available at: https://www2.gov.bc.ca/gov/content/health/accessing-health-care/home-community-care/are-you-eligible [accessed 23.10.22].

Busby, C. (2021) 'Home care spending data are a launching point for better policies', Ottawa: Policy Options. Available at: https://policyoptions.irpp.org/magazines/november-2021/home-care-spending-data-are-a-launching-point-for-better-policies/ [accessed 21.02.23].

Canadian Institute of Health Information (CIHI). (2010) 'Home care'. Available at: https://www.cihi.ca/en/home-care [accessed 01.08.22].

Deloitte. (2020) 'COVID-19: Virtual care is here to stay', Toronto: Deloitte LLP. Available at: https://www2.deloitte.com/content/dam/Deloitte/ca/Documents/life-sciences-health-care/ca-covid-19-digital-health-and-virtual-care-aoda-en.pdf [accessed 21.02.23].

Eales, J., Fast, J., Boger, J. and the DATcares team. (2017) 'Designing technology that cares: barriers to carers' technology adoption'. Available at: https://rapp.ualberta.ca/wp-content/uploads/sites/49/2019/07/Barriers-to-Carers-Technology-Adoption-DATcares-research-brief-compressed.pdf [accessed on 30.11.22].

Eales, J., Fast, J., Duncan, K. and Keating, N. (2022) 'Value of Family Carers in Canada'. *Research on Aging, Policies and Practice Working Paper*. Edmonton, AB: AGEWELL.

Fast, J., Lero, D., DeMarco, R., Ferreira, H. and Eales, J. (2014) 'Combining care work and paid work: is it sustainable?' Edmonton, AB: Research on Aging, Policies and Practice.

Gilmore, H. (2018) 'Unmet home care needs in Canada', Ottawa, ON: Statistics Canada. Available at: https://www150.statcan.gc.ca/n1/pub/82-003-x/2018011/article/00002-eng.pdf [accessed 21.02.23].

Government of Canada. (2017) 'Canada reaches health funding agreement with the Northwest Territories, Nunavut and Yukon'. Available at: https://www.canada.ca/en/health-canada/news/2017/01/canada-reaches-health-funding-agreement-northwest-territories-nunavut-yukon.html [accessed 23.10.22].

Government of the Northwest Territories. (2020) 'NWT home and community care review'. Available at: https://www.ntassembly.ca/sites/assembly/files/td_150-192.pdf [accessed 23.10.22].

Health PEI. (2022) 'Home care – home care program'. Available at: https://pe.211.ca/result/home-care-home-care-program-65174357 [accessed 23.10.22].

Hermus, G., Stonebridge, C., Thériault, L. and Bounajm, F. (2012) 'Home and community care in Canada: an economic footprint', Ottawa, ON: Conference Board of Canada. Available at: https://silo.tips/download/report-may-home-and-community-care-in-canada-an-economic-footprint-health-health [accessed 23.10.22].

InnoTraction Solutions Inc. (2009) 'Continuing care health technologies roadmap: aging in the right place'. Available at: https://open.alberta.ca/dataset/0ce39a94-7c58-49d5-9183-32332ed50315/resource/9b6230ea-1541-40cd-8e02-481785f905fa/download/ccht-roadmap.pdfinnot [accessed 23.10.22].

Innovation, Science and Economic Development Canada. (2019a) 'High-speed access for all: Canada's connectivity strategy', Ottawa, ON: ISED. Available at: https://ised-isde.canada.ca/site/high-speed-internet-canada/en/canadas-connectivity-strategy/high-speed-access-all-canadas-connectivity-strategy [accessed 21.02.23].

Innovation, Science and Economic Development Canada. (2019b) 'Rural opportunity, national prosperity: an economic development strategy for rural Canada', Ottawa: ISED. Available at: https://ised-isde.canada.ca/site/rural/en/rural-opportunity-national-prosperity-economic-development-strategy-rural-canada [accessed 21.02.23].

Johnson, C.S., Bacsu, J., McIntosh, T., Jeffery, B. and Novik, N. (2017) 'Home care in Canada: an environmental scan'. Regina, SK: Saskatchewan Population Health and Evaluation Research Unit, University of Regina and University of Saskatchewan. Available at: https://spheru.ca/publications/files/HomeCare_complexCare_environmental%20Scan18Oct2017.pdf [accessed 21.02.23].

Kaminski, J. (2021) 'The rise of tele-health: COVID-19 and beyond', *Canadian Journal of Nursing Informatics*, 16(1).

Kirby, M. (2005) 'The health of Canadians – the federal role'. Available at: https://health.gov.on.ca/en/public/programs/lhin/docs/hcc_report.pdf [accessed 23.10.22].

Leone, C., Lim, J.S.L., Stern, A., Charles, J., Black, S. and Baecker, R. (2018) 'Communication technology adoption among older adult veterans: the interplay of social and cognitive factors', *Aging & Mental Health*, 22(12): 1666–1677.

Leslie, M., Gray, R.P., Eales, J., Fast, J., Magnaye, A. and Khayatzadeh-Mahani, A. (2020) 'The care capacity goals of family carers and the role of technology in achieving them', *BMC Geriatrics*, 20: doi:10.1186/s12877-020-1455-x.

Liu, L., Cruz, A.M., Ruptash, R., Barnard, S. and Juzwishin, C. (2017) 'Acceptance of global positioning system (GPS) technology among dementia clients and family caregivers', *Journal of Technology in Human Services*, 35(2): 99–119.

Lukey, A., Johnston, S., Montesanti, S., Donnelly, C., Wankah, P., Breton, M., et al (2021) 'Facilitating integration through team-based primary healthcare: a cross-case policy analysis of four Canadian provinces', *International Journal of Integrated Care*, 21(S2):12.

Mortenson, W. B., Sixsmith, A. and Beringer, R. (2016) 'No place like home? Surveillance and what home means in old age', *Canadian Journal on Aging / La Revue canadienne du vieillissement*, 35(1): 103–114.

Northwest Territories Health and Social Services Authority [NTHSSA]. (2022) 'Eligibility and how to access services'. Available at: https://www.nthssa.ca/sites/nthssa/files/resources/home_care_jmedit_0.pdf [accessed 23.10.22].

Nunavut government. (2022) 'Home and continuing care'. Available at: https://www.gov.nu.ca/information/home-and-continuing-care [accessed 23.10.22].

Ontario Government. (2015) 'Bringing care home: report of the expert group on home & community care'. Available at: https://health.gov.on.ca/en/public/programs/lhin/docs/hcc_report.pdf [accessed 18.01.23].

Ontario Telemedicine Network. (2023). Virtual Care in Action. Available at: https://otn.ca/virtual-care-in-action-archives [accessed 27.01.23].

Owens, B. (2018) 'Telemedicine on the rise but lagging in Canada', *CMAJ: Canadian Medical Association journal / Journal de l'Association médicale canadienne*, 190(38): E1149–E1150.

Pang, H., Zhao, G., Kithulegoda, N., Agarwal, P. and Ivers, N. (2022) 'Aligning virtual care in Canada with the needs of older adults', *Canadian Journal on Aging / La Revue canadienne du vieillissement*, 41(4): 641–646: doi:10.1017/S0714980821000623.

Romanow, R. (2002) 'Royal Commission on the future of health care in Canada.' Available at: https://en.wikipedia.org/wiki/Royal_Commission_on_the_Future_of_Health_Care_in_Canada [accessed 23.10.22].

Saskatchewan.ca. (n.d.) 'Individualized funding for home care'. Available at: https://www.saskatchewan.ca/residents/health/accessing-health-care-services/care-at-home-and-outside-the-hospital/individualized-funding-for-home-care#step-2 [accessed 23.10.22].

Social Supports NB. (2022) 'Long term care program'. Available at: https://socialsupportsnb.ca/en/program/long-term-care-program [accessed 23.10.22].

Starblanket, D. and Legare, M. (2019) 'Testing locally developed language apps to reduce caregiver stress and promote "aging in place" as it relates to dementia in indigenous populations', *Alzheimer's & dementia: the journal of the Alzheimer's Association*, 15(7): P145.

Starblanket, D., O'Connell, M., Gould, B., Jardine, M., Ferguson, M. and Bourassa, C. (2019) 'Defining technology user needs of indigenous older adults requiring dementia care', *Gerontechnology*, 18: 142–155.

Statistics Canada. (2020) 'Caregivers in Canada, 2018'. Available at: https://www150.statcan.gc.ca/n1/daily-quotidien/200108/dq200108a-eng.htm [accessed 23.10.22].

Statistics Canada. (2022) 'Population estimates quarterly, Q1 2022'. Available at: https://www150.statcan.gc.ca/t1/tbl1/en/tv.action?pid=1710000901 [accessed 23.10.22].

Thomas, N., Ault, L., Goubran, R., Wallace, B., Knoefel, F. and Kaye, J. (2020) 'Developing feedback methods for caregivers of persons with cognitive impairment using a home-based sensing and computing system', *Alzheimer's & Dementia*, 16(Suppl 7): e045940.

Welch, V., Mathew, C.M., Babelmorad, P., Li, Y., Ghogomu, E.T., Borg, J., Conde, M., et al (2021) 'Health, social care and technological interventions to improve functional ability of older adults living at home: an evidence and gap map', *Campbell Systematic Reviews*, 17: doi:10.1002/cl2.1175.

Xiong, C., Astell, A., Mihailidis, A. and Colantonio, A. (2018) 'Needs and preferences for technology among Chinese family caregivers of persons with dementia: a pilot study', *Journal of Rehabilitation and Assistive Technologies Engineering*, 5: 1–12.

Xiong, C., Ye, B., Mihailidis, A., Cameron, J., Astell, A., Nalder, E. and Colantonio, A. (2020) 'Sex and gender differences in technology needs and preferences among informal caregivers of persons with dementia', *BMC Geriatrics*, 20: 176.

Xiong, C., D'Souza, A. El-Khechen-Richandi, G., Mihailidis, A., Cameron, J., Astell, A., et al (2022) 'Perceptions of technology experiences and development among family caregivers and technology researchers: a qualitative study', *JMIR Formative Research*, 6 (1): e19967.

Yukon.ca. (2022) 'Learn about the home care program'. Available at: https://yukon.ca/en/health-and-wellness/care-services/learn-about-home-care-program [accessed 23.10.22].

SIX

Designing a future in longevity societies: integrating long-term care and technology-based services in Japan

Tomoko Wakui

Long-term care in Japan: policy, debates and evidence

Long-term care insurance in Japan

The Japanese Long-term Care Insurance Program (J-LTCI) – a public Long-Term Care Insurance (LTCI) programme – was introduced in 2000 to provide comprehensive support in the policy areas of long-term care, healthcare, preventive care and housing. The key focus of this reform programme is to ensure ageing in place and to provide sustainable and community-oriented care services for older adults. J-LTCI is financed in part by social insurance premiums, general taxation and co-payments, and provides only care services as opposed to cash allowances. The J-LTCI budget is made up of 50 per cent premiums paid by those aged over 40 and 50 per cent taxes (25 per cent of this from the national government, 12.5 per cent from the prefecture and 12.5 per cent from the municipality); people using services pay a co-payment of between 10 and

30 per cent and the remainder is covered by the J-LTCI budget (Yamada and Arai, 2020). The LTCI system is regulated in that only publicly certified providers – 'local governments, quasi-public welfare corporations, non-profit organizations, hospitals and for-profit companies licensed and supervised by a prefectural government' (Peng and Yeandle, 2017: 16) – are permitted to provide care.

The Japanese Long-Term Care (LTC) system uses both a needs-tested and a means-tested funding model to determine eligibility and costs for service users. Those aged 65 and over are covered by J-LTCI, but those aged 40 to 64 years are also eligible if they require care due to age-related diseases (for example, cancer, stroke, rheumatoid arthritis). When an older adult requires care, they undergo a needs assessment that considers their medical history, including physical and cognitive conditions, as well as their ability to undertake both basic and instrumental activities of daily living through a questionnaire based on activities of daily living (Tsutsui and Muramatsu, 2005; Yamada and Arai, 2020). The final decision is made by a LTC approval board, drawing on the initial assessment, a home-visit report and a medical doctor's report (Yamada and Arai, 2020). There are seven levels of long-term care that receive support via the J-LTCI: support levels 1 and 2 and care need levels 1 to 5 (least to most disabled) (Yamada and Arai, 2020). Once assessed, in-home services, day care services, preventive services and facility services are provided based on these certified levels of care needs. Care recipients are also subject to a means test that determines the level of co-payment (between 10 and 30 per cent of the total cost of the services that they use) (Ministry of Health, Labour and Welfare, 2016). Each older person in need of LTC is usually allocated a care manager who helps to make a care plan for the necessary services depending on the level of care required. Services available include home visits, bathing, rehabilitation, preventive care, LTC, care management counselling, leasing assistive devices (for example, wheelchairs, slope, handrails, cane) and home improvement.

Policy challenges

Population ageing and the demand for long-term care

The total Japanese population began to decrease in 2010; however, the proportion of those aged over 65 is increasing. In 2021, 28.9 per cent of the population (36.2 million people) were aged over 65, with this proportion forecasted to reach 38 per cent by 2055 (National Institute of Population and Social Security Research, 2017; Cabinet Office Japan, 2021b).

This rapid ageing of the population raises concerns regarding how Japan can bear the cost of social welfare and secure the human resources necessary for older adults in need of care and support. Figure 6.1 shows the rising numbers of people certified as needing support and care via J-LTCI, while Figure 6.2 demonstrates the population pyramid in 2015, 2025 and 2050 in Japan.

LTC needs typically increase when older adults reach 75 years old and as such, the proportion of older adults with care needs drastically increases from 4.2 per cent of those aged between 65 and 74 years to 31.3 per cent of those aged 75 years and older (Ministry of Health, Labour and Welfare, 2017a). Indeed, Figure 6.1 shows the number of older people requiring support and care since the introduction of J-LTCI – those aged 75 years and over account for the greatest proportion of people requiring care. Concerns regarding LTC are becoming more serious as the baby-boomer generation reaches 75 years old in 2025. The percentage of the population over 75 years old will be 17.8 per cent in 2025 and is expected to reach 23.7 per cent in 2050 as shown in Figure 6.2 (National Institute of Population and Social Security Research, 2017). The increase of those aged between 65 and 74 is moderate, while the increase of those aged over 75 is estimated to grow rapidly. These changes to Japan's population and the corresponding rise in the demand for care has, in turn, increased pressure on the LTC system. When the J-LTCI was introduced in 2000, 2.5 million older people were certified as needing care, equivalent to 14

Figure 6.1: Number of people certified as needing long-term care and support ('primary insured people') in Japan 2000–2022

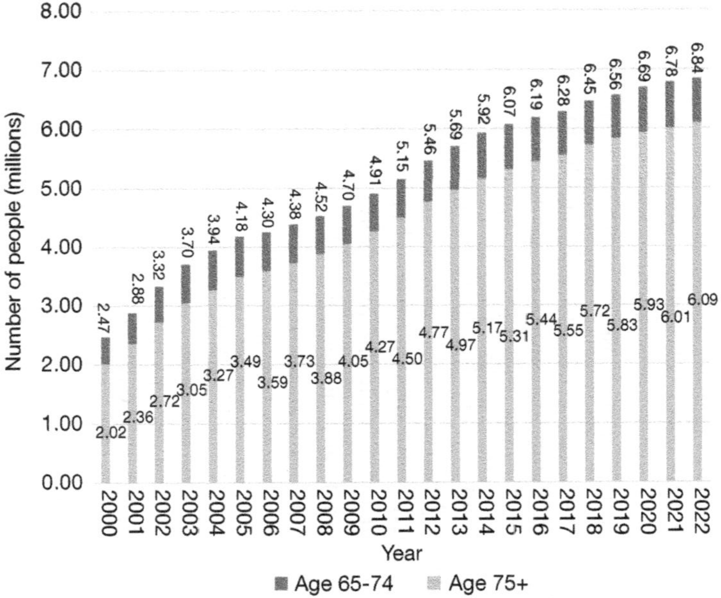

Note: Light grey shows 65–74 years old and dark grey shows 75 years and older. Data from 2000 to 2020 are definitive; from 2021 onwards are provisional.

Source: Report Survey on Situation of Long-term Care Insurance Service by Ministry of Health, Labour and Welfare (Japan) (2022)

Figure 6.2: Changes in Japanese population structure in 2015, 2025 and 2050

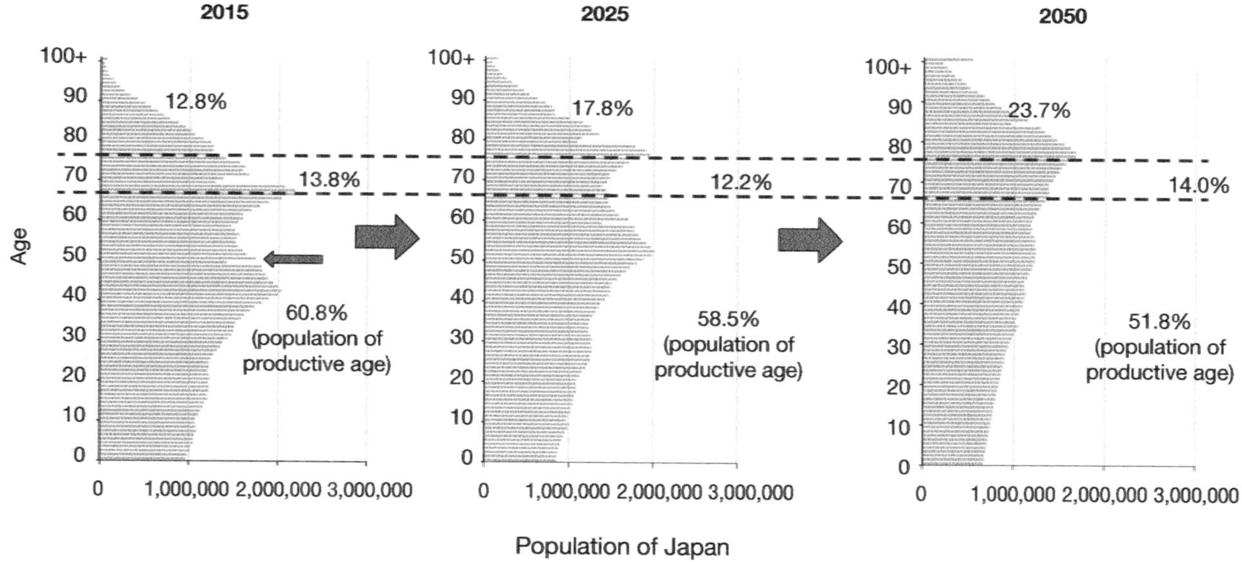

Source: National Institute of Population and Social Security Research (2017), and Cabinet Office Japan (2021b)

per cent of the older adult population, which had increased to 6.76 million older adults (19 per cent) by 2021 (Ministry of Health, Labour and Welfare, 2001, 2021). This figure is expected to increase further as the population continues to age. Such increased demand on the LTC system raises grave and urgent concerns about its sustainability.

Changing family norms and structures

Before Japan introduced J-LTCI, most older adults with care needs had been traditionally supported by families with limited public services. The introduction of the mandatory J-LTCI shifted this focus. While in the programme's infancy there was some reluctance in taking up services, the services are now widely available as a right of older people who need care. Within families, women typically shouldered most of the caregiving responsibilities (Traphagan and Knight, 2003). This kin-based care arrangement arose because women, at this time, were few in paid employment and the dominant type of household was multi-generational, including older adults with care needs. As such, 'female homemakers' – wives or daughters-in-law of older adults in households – provided LTC to older parents-in-law or spouses.

However, the number of women engaging in paid employment outside of the home has been gradually increasing, shifting their focus away from the traditional role of family caregiver. The female employment rate rose from 45.7 per cent in 1975 to 53.2 per cent in 2021 (Statistics Bureau of Japan; Ministry of Internal Affairs and Communications Japan, 2022). In addition, the preference for three-generational households has declined. Two decades ago, half of all households in Japan that included older adults with care needs were multi-generational, but this proportion decreased to 20 per cent in 2013 (Ministry of Health, Labour and Welfare, 2019). Correspondingly, 22.9 per cent of care recipients were found to be living alone at home (compared with less than 5 per cent in 1992), and older couple households increased to 22.0 per cent by 2013 from 15.0 per cent in 1989 (Ministry of Health, Labour and Welfare, 2019; Wakui, 2018). The numbers of older adults living alone or with partners are also expected to increase further in line with wider age-related demographic shifts (Cabinet Office Japan, 2021a). In addition, the numbers of older people needing care with unmarried children have gradually increased. These changes are influenced by a change in norms and preferences related to multi-generational living arrangements, with three-generational households reducing in prevalence; the rapid decline in marriage rates for both men and women; and the reduced birth rate (Wakui, 2018).

These changes to family and household formations in Japan have implications for how older adults age in place. Currently, around 80 per cent of older care recipients live in community settings, either their own homes or with families, with the remaining 20 per cent living in residential care settings (Cabinet Office Japan, 2021a). Many of those who live outside of residential care facilities are supported by families using J-LTCI (Cabinet Office Japan, 2021a). As increasing numbers of older adults in Japan live alone, there will be a greater need for social services to support both those who need care solitary and their families within the next 20 years (Cabinet Office Japan, 2021a).

Shortage of care workers

Another issue for LTC in Japan is the supply of formal or paid care workers necessary to support older adults with care needs. It is projected that by 2025, there will be a shortage of some 337,000 care workers (Ministry of Health, Labour and Welfare, 2018). Low wages, combined with the physical and mental demands of paid care work, have contributed to a shortage of paid care workers. In Japan, annual job turnover among paid care workers is 16.7 per cent, which is consistently higher when compared with the 11.6 per cent rate for other sectors of the economy (Ministry of Health, Labour and Welfare, 2017b). Between 50 and 80 per cent of care workers report serious back pain caused by physical strain (Takeda and Takagi, 2016), despite implementation of a psychosocial approach to pain prevention, including preventive exercises, risk assessment at work, and social support from co-workers and supervisors. To address the shortage of care workers in LTC, comprehensive measures have been introduced by national government, including: improving the wage levels of LTC staff; recruiting and training a diverse workforce, such as senior volunteers; promoting care work to younger students; installing information and communication technologies for operational efficiency; and acceptance of migrant care labour. Nonetheless, the rates of job vacancies in the field of LTC remain high.

Economic issues

The increasing cost of social security has consistently been an issue in ageing societies with comprehensive social welfare systems; as society ages, costs associated with pensions and also medical and LTC dramatically increase. As a proportion of Japan's Gross Domestic Product, medical costs are approaching 8 per cent and for LTC, they are around 3 per cent; both are expected to increase. In the area of medical care, the government is promoting the prevention of severe cases of diabetes; specific health check-ups and health guidance; the use of generic drugs; and optimising medical costs through the proper use of drugs. In the area of LTC, the government aims to reduce costs by improving the service infrastructure to meet local needs. Figure 6.3 shows the increasing financial pressure on society with regard to social security in Japan. The total costs of pensions, medical care and LTC have been increasing as society gets older.

Figure 6.3: Annual governmental budget for social security in Japan from fiscal year 2013 to 2022, by purpose (in trillion Japanese yen)

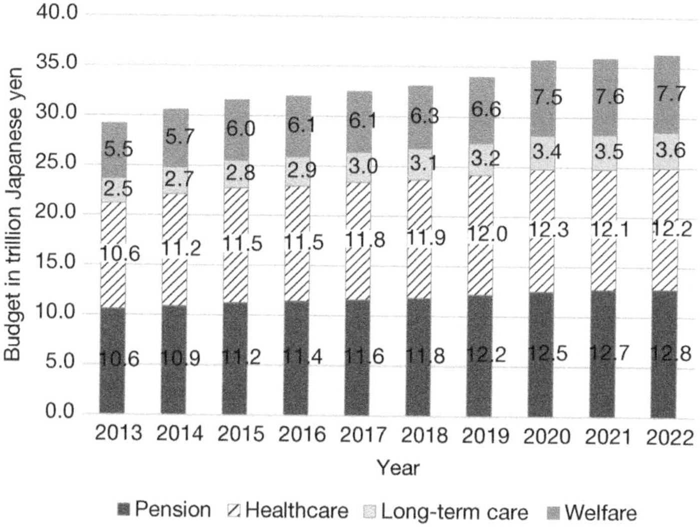

Source: Ministry of Finance Japan (2021)

Integrating technology and long-term care in an ageing society

Policy initiatives in introducing technology to long-term care

The integration of technology into LTC provision in Japan is argued to be necessary to not only secure the sustainability of the long-term insurance programme in the context of an ageing society, but also to support the rising number of single-person households. The Ministry of Health, Labour and Welfare (MHLW) and the Ministry of Economy, Trade and Industry (METI) have prioritised the development and promotion of assistive technologies around six main areas of LTC: support for 1. lifting or physically moving a person with care needs; 2. mobility; 3. bathing; 4. continence; 5. monitoring and communication; and 6. LTC operational efficiency.

METI provides a platform aiming to educate all those involved in care robots (developers, care staffs, older adults, municipalities that are care insurers, and so on) to develop and use care technology safely and effectively in care settings. The website provides various information on care technology, an initiative by the Japan Agency for Medical Research and Development (AMED) related to care robotics, care technology products, information on related seminars/events, and so on. On this website, information on products related to care robots is listed by purpose of assistance, and the status of product development (information on development in progress, commercialisation and end of production) can be checked. Therefore, care workers or LTC facility managers interested in care robots can be informed about the products. On the other hand, product developers could get information on funding to develop and introduce care technology (development assistance project), supported by the Japan Agency for Medical Research and Development, based on the social survey results of public opinions on care robots conducted by the Cabinet Office, or on other research evidence.

Technology funded by long-term care insurance

Under the current LTC insurance programme, benefits cover welfare devices for older adults with care needs, which help their activities of daily living or their functional abilities. This includes wheelchairs, walkers, handrails and ramps at home, pressure ulcer prevention equipment, lifts (excluding suspending devices), automatic excretion disposal equipment and monitoring devices in residential care institutions (Ministry of Health, Labour and Welfare, 2022). In addition, several revisions were made in the 2021 revision of LTC fees, with the aiming of improving the quality of LTC services and promoting operational efficiency through the use of technology. For example, in the case where multiple technology devices, such as monitoring devices, are installed in special nursing homes for older adults, the care staffing requirements are eased under some regulatory requirements (for example, 70 per cent or more of new residents are certified as requiring care 4 or 5, or the level of independence in daily living with dementia is somewhat severe) (Ministry of Health, Labour and Welfare, n.d.).

Care robots

Care robots are a particular area of policy focus. The definition of 'care robot' in MHLW refers to an LTC device that uses technology, including sensor system, intelligence and control systems, in order to support autonomy and independence of care recipients and reduce demands on caregivers (Ministry of Health, Labour and Welfare, n.d.). Examples include:

- the use of robotic technology to physically assist caregivers to lift and move older adults;
- a device that uses robotic technology to predict defecation and guides the user to the toilet at the appropriate moment;
- platform for devices using robotic technology with fall detection sensors or external communication functions to be used in home care;
- a device that collects and stores information associated with LTC tasks, including monitoring well-being, mobility and continence support.

Data and data analytics

The MHLW-established LIFE project (Long-term care Information system For Evidence) is a further example of government investment into technologies in LTC arrangements (Ministry of Health, Labour and Welfare, n.d.). This project is part of a policy push towards the 'science of care' that uses health- and care-related data to predict not only the decline in physical and cognitive functions, but also the necessary care services and the number of LTC workers required. There is also the aspiration that use of data in this way will improve the efficiency of care for care workers. In addition, being able to predict the necessary support needed will facilitate the planning of support for both formal and informal carers, including measures to facilitate the balance of work and caregiving, reducing the burden of caregiving caused by the unpredictability of care, preventing caregiver burnout and leading to a sustainable care system.

With these considerations in mind, the purpose of the LIFE project is to promote the practice of LTC based on scientific evidence through the collection and analysis of information from LTC-related databases. LTC facilities, including both community and institutional services, are encouraged to use LIFE, which accumulates evidence on LTC services and provides feedback. The aim is that the quality of care will be improved based on the PDCA ('Plan-Do-Check-Act') cycle model. The PDCA model is a method usually applied in business for the control and continual improvement of some processes and products (Tague, 2005). First, the 'Plan' phase includes establishing objectives and processes for desired results. The 'Do' phase is processing the improvements to the process or product. The 'Check' phase is used to evaluate the products and the process against objectives determined in the Plan phase. The final 'Act' phase is used to reformulate the process based on outcomes from the previous phases. This process is intended to promote continuous improvement with this cycle model (Tague, 2005).

The LIFE project has brought together data from two key sources since April 2021: the CHASE (Care, HeAlth, Status, and Events) system, for collecting evidence on LTC services (established in 2020) and VISIT (monitoring and evaluation for rehabilitation services for LTC, established in 2017), which collects rehabilitation-related information such as plans and meeting reports from rehabilitation facilities. LIFE enables the comparison of data at both individual and institutional levels. By using LIFE, data collected from facilities nationwide are analysed and the most appropriate care plans for the individual care recipient's condition is presented, allowing care planners to quickly find what care plan is best suited for each person. The introduction of LIFE has been encouraged to allow even inexperienced care workers to provide care planning based on practical data analysis. Using LIFE may support care workers to make plans relying on not only their experiences, but also other facilities' trials and experiences. The LIFE project started operating in 2021, and in 2022, a survey and research project is planned to evaluate utilising LIFE and to verify the potential for using LIFE in home visiting services and care management services. In particular, the actual status of cooperation between multiple professions in rehabilitation/functional training, oral health, nutrition, and so on, is to be ascertained, as well as the impact on facilities and challenges related to introducing LIFE. A survey focusing on the effects and challenges of LIFE implementation is planned (Ministry of Health, Labour and Welfare, n.d.).

Recent research evidence on the use of technologies in long-term care

Technology and residential care

As shown above, the Japanese government has made some efforts to introduce technology in many ways in the LTC settings. However, in practice, technologies have not yet been well adopted in both institutional and community settings.

In 2021, the Center for Workplace Safety in Nursing Care surveyed 9,244 LTC facilities, including home care facilities, day care facilities and residential care facilities, to collect data about operational challenges, including the implementation of assistive technology and LTC robots at each facility. According to the report, only 19.4 per cent of facilities had some type of care robot, with the most common type installed for monitoring and communication (3.7 per cent of survey responses), followed by bathing assistance (1.8 per cent), lifting and transfer assistance (1.5 per cent), and lastly, systems for recording and reporting data related to care provision (1.3 per cent). Residential facilities had the highest rate of adoption, with 40 per cent introducing some types of care robot, and 16.6 per cent used robotics for monitoring people's falls, vital signs, and so on (Center for Long-Term Care Work Stability, 2020).

Current data indicates a higher rate of adoption for assistive devices compared to care robots, whereby 69 per cent had some type of assistive devices, such as a bed with a body positioning function, air mat, devices for wheelchair elevation function or mobile lifts. Residential facilities had the highest installation rate, with more than 90 per cent having installed some type of assistive devices. Among residential facilities, more than 80 per cent had a bed with a body positioning function, 83..3 per cent had wheelchair scales and 69.2 per cent had special bathtubs (for example, those that operate with a mobile lift or those that can be opened and closed on the sides) (Center for Long-Term Care Work Stability, 2020).

The Center for Workplace Safety in Nursing Care survey data (Center for Long-Term Care Work Stability, 2020) indicate the challenges in introducing or using assistive technologies in residential care settings relate to: the high installation costs (50.6 per cent), the need for wide spaces to install or store the devices (26 per cent), and the lack of benefits commensurate with the investment required (26 per cent). For the use of robotics in residential care facilities specifically, high installation costs (60.5 per cent), the lack of benefits commensurate with the investment required (4 per cent) and the concerns about malfunction (34.5 per cent) were the most cited barriers to adoption and use. There was also an interesting contrast between the responses related to feelings of discomfort in using particular devices to provide care, with a far higher proportion of those surveys reporting this was an issue for care robots compared with assistive devices (25.1 per cent compared with 6.3 per cent). The data indicate resistance over care robots is relatively higher than assistive devices; in particular, care workers feel more uncomfortable when using care robots rather than assistive devices.

Based on the above Center for Long-Term Care Work Stability (2020) report, assistive devices, such as beds, lifts or special bathtubs, may be trusted and installed as supportive devices in LTC settings, in particular, in residential care settings, even though the high installation cost can be challenging and the maintenance can be time-consuming. Concern about malfunction of devices seems to be low and resistance among care workers to utilise these assistive devices is also low. However, care workers show higher resistance for using care robots in care settings due to unfamiliarity and have greater concerns about possible malfunctioning of care robots (Center for Long-Term Care Work Stability, 2020).

Robotics and residential care

Where care robots have been used, there have been discussions about their role in replacing human care workers. For example, Ishikawa (2017) reported their experience of installing technology at an LTC facility in metropolitan Tokyo that uses several robot devices and sensors and utilises information and communications technology to improve the work environment by assisting overburdened care workers. In this facility, advanced technology and robot devices are used to monitor every movement of older residents, 24 hours a day; share care records in real time among care workers and family members; and assist care workers with transferring residents from their beds to their wheelchairs, and from their wheelchair to a toilet seat. He analysed their process of installing technology and claimed that these technologies have helped reduce physical and mental burdens on care workers (Ishikawa, 2017). However, Ishikawa emphasises that technology cannot and should not entirely replace human care. In LTC, technology should be used to assist in physically and mentally demanding tasks, thus reducing the burdens of care. Care workers must be instructed on the responsibilities best assisted with technology and how to operate the necessary devices effectively. Ishikawa (2017) proposes that with the use of technology, care workers will be able to spend more quality time with older residents and concentrate on LTC work.

However, other empirical studies of the use of robotics in residential care facilities have found that instead of increasing workforce capacity, they have a negative impact on job content and quality, and the number of tasks assigned to care workers. An ethnographic study of the use of robots in residential care facilities in Japan found that rather than replacing care workers or increasing the capacity of an already overstretched workforce, these devices instead *displaced* the staff, conducting some of the more 'hands on' care tasks while creating new demands. Wright explored the use of Paro, the robotic seal, which required care staff to supervise and 'protect' what was an expensive investment, especially when one resident learnt how to remove the seal's faux-fur skin. In this study, Wright also observed the use of Pepper, a humanoid robot, which, although advertised as an autonomous, standalone robot, required a great deal of intervention from staff. Care workers in the setting used similar language to describe their tasks and roles in relation to Pepper as with the people they cared for; Pepper was at risk of falling and 'injuring' itself, 'hard of hearing' and needed help communicating, and required staff to 'watch and protect' it. Pepper also took on tasks care staff had previously enjoyed, for example, leading the exercise classes, with care staff instead copying the moves. Wright describes this: '[t]his extra human labor has been hidden in plain sight, discounted in promotional videos, and overlooked in enthusiastic state strategy documents, but keenly felt by caregivers sensitive to any change in the flow of daily life because of the tight constraints on their time' (Wright, 2019: 348).

Older people's views of technology and care

Several studies have focused on the acceptability and use of technology by older people to support care in Japan. Our research team conducted a survey of people aged 40–79 in Japan about their use of technology to support their own care needs. Our cross-sectional study of 3,261 respondents revealed some interesting results about the acceptance of care technologies (Itoh et al, 2021). We found acceptance of care technologies differs between Basic Activities of Daily Living and Instrumental Activities of Daily Living and types of care technologies, with highest acceptance rates reported by women with higher education or income and experiences of informal caregiving (Itoh et al, 2021). The experiences of informal care may help people consider the burdensome situations of family caregiving, which may lead to a more favourable attitude toward technology in a care setting.

A study by Wakui et al (2022) using data collected in 2020 examines the relationship between people's trust in the Japanese social welfare system and acceptance of technology for activities of daily living. This survey of community-dwelling individuals aged between 40 and 89 across Japan explored their acceptance of help provided via artificial intelligence or robotics technology in five dimensions of activities of daily living, in addition to a 5-point Likert scale to assess their trust in social security. A total of 4,047 responses with a mean age of 60.6 (standard deviation=11.3) were analysed. Of those, 13.2 per cent preferred help from humans only in Activities of Daily Living, while for 86.8 per cent, the use of some assistive technology was acceptable. This study revealed that the female and younger respondents and those who had better health and had completed higher education were more likely to accept artificial intelligence or robotics technology in all/some Activities of Daily Living if they needed assistance; those with higher trust in social security, however, were less likely to accept technology (Wakui et al, 2022). This study suggests that a well-trusted insurance programme may hinder people's preference for technology to support future possible care requirements. The current environment in which older adults are able to use services when they require may not make people feel the need for technology in an alternative way.

Conclusion

Japan's demographic changes of rapid ageing and depopulation have created unforeseen challenges. The society has struggled to maintain the quality of life of people while sustaining the social system to support older adults, as well as those with care needs. The declining birth rate has led to smaller household structures; many families who traditionally supported their older adults have no longer been available. The financial burden of maintaining the public LTC and medical insurance programmes has increased gradually. The sustainability of the social system has long been debated. It is against this context that Japanese governments have promoted the use and development of technologies for use in care provision.

However, as has been discussed, adoption and use of technologies have not met the levels aspired to by governments. From the experiences in Japan on the barriers to the use and adoption of technologies in LTC, findings can be grouped into three main arguments. First, there are structural problems, such as higher installation cost, the maintenance issues or challenges related to the acquisition of skills to use technology. These structural barriers can be due to a lack of communication between the developers and the care providers who use the technology, that is, the technology services are not being provided in a way that meets caregivers' needs.

Second, studies have highlighted individuals' subjective acceptance/resistance to/against different types of technology. There is also the matter of caregivers not trusting the technology enough to invest in it (for example, time to acquire knowledge and training to use the equipment), or not having enough trust in it. In addition to technology adoption, trust in continued use is also another issue. Even though people trust a technology and start using it, the devices may require other physical and financial investment to maintain them.

The final barrier could relate to the current social security system. An area that has yet to be explored empirically is the potential of technologies to transform trust in welfare through their integration into LTC. LTC in Japan was 'socialised' fairly recently in 2000 with its separation from health and the creation of the J-LTCI. It could be argued that the creation of the J-LTCI system reflects the high level of trust the Japanese people have in their government. On the other hand, there is the possibility of transforming trust in welfare in the information society. Just as the digital divide impeded access to telehealth for groups during the COVID-19 pandemic (Chang et al, 2021), the presence of the digital divide may inhibit access to and trust in the LTC insurance programme. Issues of trust can be related to technology use in LTC; for example, if there is a disparity in the degree of adoption of LTC information and technology, it may become difficult to provide LTC support services that meet the needs of older adults, and this may lead to a change in trust in welfare. Issues of trust and technology adoption could therefore present serious problems related to the sustainability of the LTC system.

References

Cabinet Office Japan. (2021a) 'Annual report on the aging society,' White Paper. Available at: https://www8.cao.go.jp/kourei/whitepaper/w-2021/zenbun/03pdf_index.html [accessed 15.06.22].

Cabinet Office Japan. (2021b) 'Population estimation'. Available at: https://www.stat.go.jp/data/jinsui/2021np/index.html [accessed 15.06.22].

Center for Long-Term Care Work Stability. (2020) 'Survey results on care work in 2020', Center for Long-Term Care Work Stability. Available at: http://www.kaigo-center.or.jp/report/2021r01_chousa_01.html [accessed 15.06.22].

Chang, J.E., Lai, A.Y., Gupta, A., Nguyen, A.M., Berry, C.A. and Shelley, D.R. (2021). 'Rapid transition to telehealth and the digital divide: implications for primary care access and equity in a post-COVID era', *Milbank Q*, 99: 340–368.

Ishikawa, K. (2017) 'On-site reforms through the use of long-term care robots', 地域ケアリング (*Community Care*), 19: 19–24.

Itoh, S., Miwa, H., Wu, V. X., Okuyama, A., Watanabe, K., Ikeuchi, T., et al (2021) 'Acceptance of care technologies to support activities of daily living by middle-aged and older adults in Japan: a cross-sectional study', *International Journal of Nursing Studies Advances*, 3: 100042.

Ministry of Finance. (2021) 'Annual governmental budget for social security in Japan from fiscal year 2013 to 2022, by purpose (in trillion Japanese yen)'. Available at: https://www.statista.com/statistics/1214041/japan-social-security-governmental-budget-by-purpose/ [accessed 25.11.22].

Ministry of Health, Labour and Welfare. (2001) 'Annual report on status of long-term care insurance services'. Available at: https://www.mhlw.go.jp/toukei/list/84-1.html [accessed 15.06.22].

Ministry of Health, Labour and Welfare. (2016) 'Riyosya-Hutan' (in Japanese). Available at: www.mhlw.go.jp/file/05-Shingikai-12601000-Seisakutoukatsukan-Sanjikanshitsu_Shakaihoshoutantou/0000171814.pdf [accessed 15.06.22].

Ministry of Health, Labour and Welfare. (2017a) 'Annual report on status of long-term care insurance services'. Available at: http://www.mhlw.go.jp/toukei/list/84-1.html [accessed 30.07.2018].

Ministry of Health, Labour and Welfare. (2017b) 'Current situation of care work'. Available at: https://www.mhlw.go.jp/content/12602000/000482541.pdf [accessed 15.06.22].

Ministry of Health, Labour and Welfare. (2018) 第7期介護保険事業計画に基つ゛く介護人材の必要数について (Concerning the required number of care staff based on the 7th Long Term Care Insurance Plan). Available at: https://www.mhlw.go.jp/stf/houdou/0000207323.html [accessed 27.01.23].

Ministry of Health, Labour and Welfare. (2019) 'Comprehensive survey of living conditions'. Available at: https://www.mhlw.go.jp/english/database/db-hss/cslc-index.html [accessed 15.06.22].

Ministry of Health, Labour and Welfare. (2021) 'Annual report on status of long-term care insurance services'. Available at: https://www.mhlw.go.jp/toukei/list/84-1.html [accessed 15.06.22].

Ministry of Health, Labour and Welfare (2022) 'Welfare devices under long-term care insurance program'. Available at: https://www.mhlw.go.jp/stf/seisakunitsuite/bunya/0000212398.html [accessed 18.07.22].

Ministry of Health, Labour and Welfare. (n.d.) 'Long-term care information system for evidence'. Available at: https://www.mhlw.go.jp/stf/shingi2/0000198094_00037.html [accessed 15.06.22].

Ministry of Health, Labour and Welfare. (n.d.) 'Promoting the development and dissemination of long-term care robots'. Available at: https://www.mhlw.go.jp/stf/seisakunitsuite/bunya/0000209634.html [accessed 16.06.22].

National Institute of Population and Social Security Research. (2017) 'Population estimation in Japan'. Available at: https://www.ipss.go.jp/pp-zenkoku/j/zenkoku2017/pp29_gaiyou.pdf [accessed 15.06.22].

Peng, I. and Yeandle, S.M. (2017) *Eldercare Policies in East Asia and Europe: Mapping Policy Changes and Variations and Their Implications*. UN Women Discussion Paper Series, New York: UN Women.

Statistics Bureau of Japan; Ministry of Internal Affairs and Communications (Japan). (2022) 'Percentage of people in the labor force among total population aged 15 years and older in Japan from 1973 to 2021, by gender'. Available at: https://www.stat.go.jp/data/roudou/longtime/zuhyou/lt03-06.xlsx [accessed 15.06.22].

Tague, N. R. (2005) *The Quality Toolbox* (2nd edition), Milwaukee, WI: ASQ Quality Press.

Takeda, K. and Takagi, N. (2016) 'Back pain of care workers: comparison based on years of experience', 介護福祉士 (Care Worker), 20/21: 90–102.

Traphagan, J.W. and Knight, J. (2003) *Demographic Change and the Family in Japan's Aging Society*, Albany, New York: State University of New York Press.

Tsutsui, T. and Muramatsu, N. (2005) 'Care-needs certification in the long-term care insurance system of Japan', *Journal of the American Geriatrics Society*, 53(3): 522–527.

Wakui, T. (2018) 'Variety of caregiving arrangement and future long-term care system in Japan', *Japanese Journal of Gerontology*, 40: 301–307.

Wakui, T., Itoh, S., Miwa, H., Ikeuchi, T. and Watanabe, K. (2022) 'Does trust in social security inhibit acceptance of assistive technology for ADL help?' Presented at Gerontological Society of America 2022 Annual Scientific Meeting, Indiana, USA.

Wright, J. (2019) 'Robots vs migrants? Reconfiguring the future of Japanese institutional eldercare', *Critical Asian Studies*, 51(3): 331–354.

Yamada, M. and Arai, H. (2020) 'Long-term care system in Japan', *Annals of Geriatric Medicine and Research*, 24(3): 174.

SEVEN

Care technologies for ageing societies: key lessons

Matthew Lariviere and Kate Hamblin

This volume has provided insight into the role of technologies in care provision in five nations from across the globe. Though these nations have very different policy legacies and frameworks, and expectations and norms related to care, they face similar challenges due to the ageing of their populations. All five countries have in policy and/or practice explored the various ways technologies can support the sustainability – in largely economic terms only – of their care provision. Here, we will provide a brief synthesis of the material covered in the preceding five chapters covering each nation. We will highlight how and to what extent the role of technologies converges and diverges within and across international care systems, and to what effect. We close with: a brief summary of the main issues related to each country; the key areas of convergence and divergence; and recommendations for policy, practice and further research.

Brief summary of key points from each country

In **England**, technology in social care arrangements emerged with alarm systems in the 1960s and was initially used to facilitate 'ageing in place' and discharge from clinical settings by managing risks (Fisk, 2003). In the past ten years, technology has been presented in policy discourse as a solution to a 'crisis' facing social care and a way to contain costs, staff resources and improve quality. England has seen a variety of top-down funding opportunities for service development and pilots by local authorities. This, when combined with the lack of a 'blueprint' or a requirement that every local authority provides technology-enabled care services, has resulted in uneven practice.[1] There are examples of local authorities using these funding schemes to explore digital technologies and systems in care provision, including platforms, artificial intelligence (AI), robotics and the 'smarter' use of data, as well as programmes to improve the information and communications technology (ICT) infrastructure and connectivity, thereby fixing issues 'further up the line'. The COVID-19 pandemic accelerated adoption in practice but again, this has been patchy and uneven. There was also investment in developing the evidence base related to technology and care in the hope that practice would catch up with policy rhetoric. However, the picture painted by the resultant research was not as overwhelmingly positive as perhaps hoped by policy makers.

The chapter on **Australia** explored the significant reform of care systems and services in 2013 with the move towards a consumer-directed care (CDC) model to facilitate older adults to 'age in place'. Research presented in this volume has highlighted the resultant long waiting lists, inadequate funding and a lack of flexibility from this system reform. These reforms were, however, allied with the promotion of technologies by Australian governments to support 'ageing in place' by allowing for home care packages for older adults to be spent on assistive technologies, typically to support activities of daily living, mobility and communication in addition to telehealth devices.

As with England, there are debates in Australia regarding the evidence base related to technology and care in terms of both the quality and quantity of research available. The chapter's authors in response developed three research studies to explore policy frameworks for the delivery of technology and care, their outcomes for older adults, how they are used by health professionals in practice to support people to age in place, and the barriers to their adoption. With regard to the latter, a key issue highlighted by the authors' work and the COVID-19 pandemic was the importance of digital literacy in mediating the outcomes of technology. The authors highlight the centrality and possibilities of partnership working and greater co-design of technologies and services to ensure their use and appropriateness.

The **German** long-term care (LTC) system has a strong subsidiarity principle that is a point of tension with an ageing population and women's increased labour force participation, which alter the demand and supply of traditional care provision. As with England and Australia, policy discourse has emphasised the potential of technologies to support the provision of care and reduce demands on an overstretched system and overburdened carers. Germany adopted a social insurance-based LTC system, payment from which older adults can purchase specific types of technologies. A further point of tension is therefore between the policy aspirations as exemplified in expert-led documents such as the 8th Ageing Report and their curtailment in practice by rules regarding which technologies are available for purchase via long-term care insurance. Research has highlighted in the German context the importance of digital connectivity and skills in facilitating the use of technologies in care arrangements, and that other intersectionalities alongside a person's age are a factor that affects access and adoption of such technologies.

Canada does not have a national social care system per se, with instead provision devolved to provinces, to territories and, for some groups, by the federal governance. Provision is typically needs- and means-tested and this extends to the provision of technology used in care arrangements. The devolved nature of provision means that there is variation across Canada, both in terms of the types of technologies and services available and whether these are provided directly by provinces, can be purchased using a monthly stipend or are self-funded. Private companies are leading the drive towards the use of technologies in care, focusing on four main areas: 1. care management/coordination; 2. smart homes; 3. outdoor tracking; and 4. communication technologies. Although the majority of care in Canada is provided by unpaid carers, there is very limited provision either by private developers or the provinces of technologies to support this group. Digital connectivity is a particular issue that affects the use of technologies in care arrangements in Canada and, in response, policies focused on delivering high-speed broadband have been announced. The emergence of the federally funded AGE-WELL National Centre of Excellence has demonstrated technology as a key priority for the Canadian government for the care of older Canadians and commercial opportunities for the Canadian economy.

In response to a rapidly ageing population, **Japan's** governments have prioritised the development of technologies for use in care settings, with a particular focus on: 1. lifting or physically moving a person with care needs; 2. mobility; 3. bathing; 4. continence; 5. monitoring and communication; and 6. LTC operational efficiency. Funding programmes have focused on the development of robots for particular use in residential care settings. In practice, however, the use of such technology is limited to a relatively small proportion of residential care homes, reflecting their high costs and practical issues, such as storage and manoeuvrability. The high costs and practical issues with the provision of technology in care settings echoes similar facets identified in England.

Divergence and convergence

A clear area of divergence between the countries selected was their very different **care systems** (or their absence) with responsibility for local and national care provision. Despite the advent of social (care) services within many countries in the 20th century, concise and consistent definitions of publicly provided or funded care provision still evade comparative policy research. Anttonen and Sipilä's (1996) earlier attempts to identify a model to compare social care services relied on Esping-Andersen's (1990) welfare regime typology and definitions of what was then called 'personal social services' in the UK. They have argued social care services were a 'domain within which organized services are aimed at strengthening the autonomy most especially of women' and 'people who use services, such as frail elderly people and disabled people' (Anttonen and Sipilä, 1996: 90). Contemporary policy and legislation have slightly altered the focus of state care systems. In England, there is an increased presence of private and charitable providers of support services, organisations that would have been excluded from Anttonen and Sipilä's approach, which focused on state-provided services. Within this volume, it was apparent each national case referred to 'care systems' based on localised concepts and traditions to framing care provision. The volume has described such localised approaches to technology in care within a social care system (England), LTC systems (Germany and Japan), an aged care system (Australia) and the integration of social services in wider healthcare systems rather than a distinctive social care system (Canada). Each of these national contexts has highlighted distinctive forms of care provision, market actors, funding settlements and costs to the public and service users. However, they are united in their vision to support older people.

Despite very different policy and legislative contexts, there are several areas of convergence among the countries included in this volume. A key area that several countries held in common relates to the design of national care provision systems and how these designs created **internal diversity and fragmentation**. In England, Canada and Australia, technology and care provision are variable due to the devolved governance structures for care delivery, with differences in services and devices available across local authorities (England), provinces (Canada) and states and territories (Australia). As predominantly anglophone countries typified as 'liberal welfare regimes' (Esping-Andersen, 1990), such congruence of system fragmentation may further evidence the formation of liberalised 'care regimes' (Bettio and Plantenga, 2004).

Looking to areas of commonality in the guiding principles behind the use of technology in care provision, in each of the five previous chapters, this has been rationalised in policy discourses as a means to ensure **sustainability** in the face of challenges related to changing population dynamics. All countries included are facing shifting demographics, argued by policy makers to necessitate changes to the provision of care, including through the use of technology. However, technology across all countries included is being used as a tool to support the economic sustainability of social care provision, but wider discussions of environmental (the impact of producing and decommissioning digital devices, for example) and social sustainability (beyond questions around what care tasks could be replaced by technologies) are underexplored. In some countries, there is recognition that technologies could also support people providing care, either as care workers or unpaid carers, but this is comparatively limited or emergent, and therefore, so in turn are explorations as to their potential in creating socially sustainable care arrangements.

In all countries, it is also apparent that the use of technology in care is also related to the **'ageing in place' agenda** (Phillips et al, 2010), whereby the aim of policy is to enable older people to remain in or return to their homes for as long as possible, instead of moving into residential care. This policy aim has been argued to both reflect the wishes of older adults, who do not want to enter LTC facilities, and reduce costs related to the alternative provision in such facilities that would rise exponentially as populations age. However, a potential consequence is that technologies designed and delivered to support people to age in place focus on risk, rather than supporting other outcomes such as well-being and social engagement outside the home. Developments in technologies and a recognition in policy terms of the importance of well-being globally (Austin, 2020) could be a potential means to create technology and care services that address a wider agenda.

Technology is also part of increasingly marketised social care arrangements in the five countries, where choice is promoted through the use of 'personal budgets', or payments that the recipient can then spend with varying degrees of **choice and control**. It is, however, apparent that choice regarding technology is often circumscribed within pre-defined 'menus' of approved products and services that sometimes, as in the case of Germany in particular, belie the wider range of options and more innovative devices articulated in the national policy aspirations. Choice and technologies are also restricted by other practical issues, such as the **digital divide** in access to devices or adequate digital connectivity, or the skills and confidence to use technologies, which are subjects that policy in England, Canada and Germany is attempting to address. In these countries, there are examples of national-level policies to address problems related to uneven broadband connectivity.

A further area of convergence across the chapters is related to **empirical evidence** of the efficacy of technology in delivering positive outcomes in care. Evidence bases are nascent (Canada and Japan) or conflictual (England and Australia) but have been the focus of investment by governments in several of the nations (England, Canada, Germany and Japan). This investment reflects a desire in these countries to encourage the wider use of technologies in practice to support the sustainability of care provision, the assumption being that research findings demonstrating cost savings, enhanced well-being and other positive outcomes will persuade practitioners and commissioners to embed technologies in their practice. Perhaps the absence of this evidence base has contributed to the lack of scalable solutions that utilise technology to meet the challenges facing care systems; arguably none of the countries included in this book has created a wholly successful system or model of technology and care that is being delivered on a national scale, despite policy rhetoric and investment.

The country-specific analyses of policy, practice and empirical research presented in the previous five chapters have also highlighted how the COVID-19 pandemic has continued to result in increased proliferation of technology within care. Such results echo recent research findings where COVID-19 has required difficult, agile responses from care providers to continue to offer services in the context of decreased capacity, staff illness, and little preparation for such sweeping digital transformation (Puli et al, 2021).

Recommendations

Based on the insights from the policy, practice and research evidence from these five nations, we propose the following recommendations for policy makers, practitioners and researchers.

Policy makers and practitioners

- Progress requires both a clear strategic vision related to technology and care and a means to address the mismatch between national aspirations and fragmented delivery in practice.
- Balance economic aspirations with the reality of technology. While digital technology continues to be a priority for its commercial value and perception of modernisation, technology used to support older adults must ensure it meets prescribed outcomes that extend beyond cost savings.
- Policy should not identify 'technology as a solution'. Technology shapes systems and arrangements of care composed of service users, families, and care workers within complex inter- and intraorganisational contexts. Technology should be assessed critically based on service and service user preferences and agreed outcomes.

- For care provision to be sustainable, the well-being of all stakeholders is important. Greater consideration of how technologies could support both paid and unpaid carers, as well as those they support *at the same time* is important for creating care arrangements that are socially sustainable.

Researchers: academics and developers

- Debates around evidence quality shift focus away from the perspective of those using technologies in care provision, both receiving and providing care. Centring their desired outcomes, perspectives and experiences is key to developing technologies and associated services that are firstly used (as opposed to abandoned or misused) and secondly that contribute to good-quality care.
- For developers, this engagement with people receiving and providing care in the design process is crucial in ensuring products are both useful and usable by their target audiences.
- New technologies being used in care provision and arrangements will inevitably change existing professional care roles and create new ones; exploring the quality of these roles is important.
- Developments in technology and care will also need consideration of issues related to emerging ethical issues and potentially new standards and regulation.

With these recommendations, we hope that this book can help to foster a new series of priorities to embed across government, industry, care provision and academia. We must all work together to ensure future technology can support us, as a species, as societies continue to age globally.

Note

1 There are standards related to 'social alarm systems' and 'alarm receiving centres', for example, but local authorities are not required in the first instance to include technology-enabled care services as part of social care provision.

References

Anttonen, A. and Sipilä, J. (1996) 'European social care services: Is it possible to identify models?', *Journal of European Social Policy*, 6(2): 87–100.

Austin, A. (2020) *A Universal Declaration of Human Well-being*, New York: Springer International Publishing.

Bettio, F. and Plantenga, J. (2004) 'Comparing care regimes in Europe', *Feminist economics*, 10(1): 85–113.

Esping-Andersen, G. (1990) *The Three Worlds of Welfare Capitalism*, Princeton, New Jersey: Princeton University Press.

Fisk, M.J. (2003) *Social Alarms to Telecare: Older People's Services in Transition*, Bristol: Policy Press.

Phillips, J.E., Ajrouch, K.J. and Hillcoat-Nallétamby, S. (2010) *Key Concepts in Social Gerontology*, New York: Sage.

Puli, L., Layton, N., Mont, D., Shae, K., Calvo, I., Hill, K.D., et al (2021) 'Assistive technology provider experiences during the COVID-19 pandemic', *International Journal of Environmental Research and Public Health*, 18(19): 10477.

Index

References to figures appear in *italic* type; those in **bold** type refer to tables and boxes. References to endnotes show both the page number and the note number (65n1).

Q

R

S

Printed and bound by CPI Group (UK) Ltd, Croydon, CR0 4YY

15/09/2026

14962385-0001